Endoluminal Therapy for Esophageal Disease

Guest Editor

HERBERT C. WOLFSEN, MD

GASTROINTESTINAL ENDOSCOPY CLINICS OF NORTH AMERICA

www.giendo.theclinics.com

Consulting Editor
CHARLES J. LIGHTDALE, MD

January 2010 • Volume 20 • Number 1

SAUNDERS an imprint of ELSEVIER, Inc.

W.B. SAUNDERS COMPANY
A Division of Elsevier Inc.

1600 John F. Kennedy Blvd. • Suite 1800 • Philadelphia, Pennsylvania 19103-2899

http://www.giendo.theclinics.com

GASTROINTESTINAL ENDOSCOPY CLINICS OF NORTH AMERICA Volume 20, Number 1
January 2010 ISSN 1052-5157, ISBN-13: 978-1-4377-1912-3

Editor: Kerry Holland
Developmental Editor: Donald Mumford

Gastrointestinal Endoscopy Clinics of North America (ISSN 1052-5157) is published quarterly by Elsevier Inc., 360 Park Avenue South, New York, NY 10010-1710. Months of issue are January, April, July, and October. Business and Editorial Offices: 1600 John F. Kennedy Blvd., Suite 1800, Philadelphia, PA, 19103-2899. Periodicals postage paid at New York, NY and additional mailing offices. Subscription prices are $290.00 per year for US individuals, $394.00 per year for US institutions, $149.00 per year for US students and residents, $320.00 per year for Canadian individuals, $481.00 per year for Canadian institutions, $405.00 per year for international individuals, $481.00 per year for international institutions, and $207.00 per year for Canadian and foreign students/residents. To receive student/resident rate, orders must be accompanied by name of affiliated institution, date of term, and the *signature* of program/residency coordinator on institution letterhead. Orders will be billed at individual rate until proof of status is received. Foreign air speed delivery is included in all *Clinics* subscription prices. All prices are subject to change without notice. **POSTMASTER:** Send address change to *Gastrointestinal Endoscopy Clinics of North America*, Elsevier Health Sciences Division, Subscription Customer Service, 3251 Riverport Lane, Maryland Heights, MO 63043. **Customer Service: 1-800-654-2452 (US). From outside the United States, call 1-314-447-8871. Fax: 1-314-447-8029. E-mail: JournalsCustomerService-usa@elsevier.com (for print support) or JournalsOnlineSupport-usa@elsevier.com (for online support).**

Reprints. For copies of 100 or more, of articles in this publication, please contact the Commercial Reprints Department, Elsevier Inc., 360 Park Avenue South, New York, NY 10010-1710. Tel. (212) 633-3812; Fax: (212) 482-1935; E-mail: reprints@elsevier.com.

Gastrointestinal Endoscopy Clinics of North America is covered in *Excerpta Medica, MEDLINE/PubMed (Index Medicus), and MEDLINE/MEDLARS.*

Printed and bound by CPI Group (UK) Ltd, Croydon, CR0 4YY

Transferred to Digital Print 2011

Contributors

CONSULTING EDITOR

CHARLES J. LIGHTDALE, MD
Professor, Department of Medicine, Columbia University Medical Center, New York,
New York

GUEST EDITOR

HERBERT C. WOLFSEN, MD
Consultant, Division of Gastroenterology and Hepatology, Mayo Clinic Florida,
Jacksonville, Florida; Professor of Medicine, Mayo Medical School, Rochester, Minnesota

AUTHORS

JACQUES J.G.H.M. BERGMAN, MD, PhD
Associate Professor, Department of Gastroenterology and Hepatology, Academic
Medical Center, University of Amsterdam, Amsterdam, The Netherlands

ROBERT A. GANZ, MD, FASGE
Associate Professor of Medicine, University of Minnesota; Chief of Gastroenterology,
Abbott-Northwestern Hospital, Minneapolis; and Minnesota Gastroenterology, PA,
Bloomington, Minnesota

BRUCE D. GREENWALD, MD
Professor of Medicine and Fellowship Program Director, Department of Medicine,
Division of Gastroenterology and Hepatology, University of Maryland School of Medicine,
Baltimore, Maryland

SETH A. GROSS, MD
Director of Advanced Endoscopy, Division of Gastroenterology, Norwalk Hospital,
Norwalk, Connecticut

KEVIN D. HALSEY, MD
Clinical Instructor, Department of Medicine, Division of Gastroenterology and Hepatology,
University of Maryland School of Medicine, Baltimore, Maryland

HARUHIRO INOUE, MD, PhD, FASGE
Professor, Digestive Disease Center, Showa University Northern Yokohama Hospital,
Yokohama, Japan

LAITH H. JAMIL, MD
Assistant Clinical Professor, David Geffen School of Medicine at UCLA; Associate Director
of Interventional Endoscopy, Cedars-Sinai Medical Center, Los Angeles, California

MAKOTO KAGA, MD
Digestive Disease Center, Showa University Northern Yokohama Hospital,
Yokohama, Japan

SHIN-EI KUDO, MD, PhD
Digestive Disease Center, Showa University Northern Yokohama Hospital, Yokohama, Japan

HITOMI MINAMI, MD
Digestive Disease Center, Showa University Northern Yokohama Hospital, Yokohama, Japan

RICHARD I. ROTHSTEIN, MD
Professor of Medicine and Surgery, Dartmouth Medical School; Chief, Section of Gastroenterology and Hepatology, Dartmouth-Hitchcock Medical Center, Lebanon, New Hampshire

YOSHITAKA SATO, MD
Digestive Disease Center, Showa University Northern Yokohama Hospital, Yokohama, Japan

DREW B. SCHEMBRE, MD, FASGE, FACG
Division of Gastroenterology, Virginia Mason Medical Center; Associate Clinical Professor of Medicine, University of Washington, Seattle, Washington

MUHAMMAD W. SHAHID, MD
Research Fellow, Division of Gastroenterology and Hepatology, Mayo Clinic Florida, Jacksonville, Florida

C. DANIEL SMITH, MD
Professor and Chair, Department of Surgery, Mayo Clinic Florida, Jacksonville, Florida

FREDERIKE G.I. VAN VILSTEREN, MD
Research Fellow, Department of Gastroenterology and Hepatology, Academic Medical Center, University of Amsterdam, Amsterdam, The Netherlands

MELINA C. VASSILIOU, MD, Med
Assistant Professor of Surgery, Department of Surgery, McGill University Health Centre, Montreal General Hospital, Montreal, Quebec, Canada

DANIEL VON RENTELN, MD
Department of Gastroenterology, Medizinische Klinik I, Klinikum, Ludwigsburg, Germany

MICHAEL B. WALLACE, MD, MPH
Professor of Medicine, Division of Gastroenterology and Hepatology, Mayo Clinic College of Medicine, Jacksonville, Florida

HERBERT C. WOLFSEN, MD
Consultant, Division of Gastroenterology and Hepatology, Mayo Clinic Florida, Jacksonville, Florida; Professor of Medicine, Mayo Clinic College of Medicine, Rochester, Minnesota

TIMOTHY A. WOODWARD, MD
Assistant Professor of Medicine, Division of Gastroenterology, Mayo Clinic College of Medicine, Jacksonville, Florida

Contents

This introductory article summarizes decades of research from many dedicated gastrointestinal endoscopists. It provides a background to Barrett esophagus (BE), exploring the risk of progression to dysplasia and esophageal adenocarcinoma. Two premalignant conditions, BE and colon adenoma, are compared, including their progression to esophageal adenocarcinoma and colon and rectal carcinoma, respectively. A comparison of the risks of surgical treatment and post-surgical complications of these cancers and of the strikingly different paradigms for their prevention is presented. The article concludes with the rationale for endoscopic treatment of Barrett disease.

Numerous endoscopic imaging modalities have been developed and introduced into clinical practice to enhance diagnostic capabilities. In the past, detection of dysplasia and carcinoma of the esophagus has been dependent on biopsies taken during standard white-light endoscopy. Recent important developments in biophonotics have improved visualization of these subtle lesions sufficiently for cellular details to be seen in vivo during endoscopy. These improvements allow diagnosis to be made in gastrointestinal endoscopy units, thereby avoiding the cost, risk, and time delay involved in tissue biopsy and resection. Chromoendoscopy, narrow-band imaging, high-yield white-light endoscopy, Fujinon intelligent color enhancement, and point enhancement such as confocal laser endomicroscopy are examples of enhanced imaging technologies that are being used in daily practice. This article reviews endoscopic-based imaging techniques for the detection of esophageal dysplasia and carcinoma from the perspective of routine clinical practice.

Advanced cancer in the esophagus is a serious and fatal disease that invades locally to deeper layers of the esophageal wall with significant risk of nodal metastasis and invasion of adjacent organs. One reliable method of avoiding this is to detect lesions at an early stage of esophageal cancer and then to resect them locally. A major advantage of endoscopic local resection is to recover a specimen for histopathologic analysis, which helps to make a clinical decision for further therapy. Endoscopic mucosal resection (EMR) and endoscopic submucosal dissection (ESD) have already been established as the techniques of endoscopic local resection. EMR includes strip-off biopsy, double-channel techniques, cap technique, EMR using a ligating device, and so on. ESD is a newly developed technique in which submucosal dissection is carried out using an electrocautery knife to acquire a single-piece specimen.

Photodynamic therapy (PDT) is a drug and device therapy using photosensitizer drugs activated by laser light for mucosal ablation. Porfimer sodium PDT has been used extensively with proven long-term efficacy and durability for the ablation of Barrett esophagus and high-grade dysplasia. and early esophageal adenocarcinoma. However, continued use is hampered by an associated stricture risk and prolonged photosensitivity (4–6 weeks). Promising single-center European studies using other forms of PDT, such as aminolevulinic acid PDT, have not been replicated elsewhere, limiting the widespread use of other forms of PDT. Future use of PDT in esophageal disease depends on the development of improved dosimetry and patient selection to optimize treatment outcomes, while minimizing adverse events and complications.

Radiofrequency ablation (RFA) is a novel and promising treatment modality for treatment of Barrett's esophagus (BE) with high-grade dysplasia or early carcinoma. RFA can be used as a single-modality therapy for flat-type mucosa or as a supplementary therapy after endoscopic resection of visible abnormalities. The treatment protocol consists of initial circumferential ablation using a balloon-based electrode, followed by focal ablation of residual Barrett's epithelium. RFA is less frequently associated with stenosis and buried glandular mucosa as are other ablation techniques and has shown to be safe and effective in the treatment of patients with BE and early neoplasia. In this article, the technical background, current clinical experience, and future prospects of RFA are evaluated.

Accumulating evidence highlights the promising results seen with endoscopic spray cryotherapy in the treatment of dysplasia associated with Barrett esophagus and esophageal carcinoma. Published studies show that the success of spray cryotherapy to eradicate Barrett high-grade dysplasia is comparable to that for other therapies, with a favourable safety profile and high levels of patient comfort. For patients with untreatable esophageal cancer, spray cryotherapy offers a therapeutic option with the potential for complete eradication in early-stage disease and palliation in advanced cases. The mechanism of tissue injury in cryotherapy is unique, with direct cytotoxic effects and ischemic effects from vascular injury. Increased tumor cell death through induction of apoptosis and immunologic effects require further study.

Heartburn is the most common symptom associated with gastroesophageal reflux disease, and life-long proton pump inhibitor therapy is often required to control symptoms. Antireflux surgery is an alternative, but there may be significant side effects and the duration of therapeutic effect is variable. Several endoscopic antireflux techniques (E-ARTs) have been developed to enhance the function of the lower esophageal sphincter or alter the structure of the angle of His with the goal of recreating or augmenting the reflux barrier. Many methods are no longer available, and some await regulatory approval. This article reviews available data for the most common E-ARTs.

The use of self-expanding metal esophageal stents has evolved dramatically over the last 20 years. Stents themselves have morphed from simple open-mesh wire devices to a variety of partially and fully covered metal and plastic protheses designed to resist in-growth and migration. Indications include grown considerably from simply palliating malignant dysphagia to the treatment of benign conditions such as refractory strictures, perforations, and fistulas, bridging tumors through neoadjuvant therapy and even serving as support for mucosal healing after ablative therapies. This article describes the current experience with esophageal stenting for malignant and benign conditions and examines new innovations in stent design and applications.

As limited as are the studies regarding peritoneal Natural Orifice Trans-Luminal Endoscopic Surgery, mediastinal transluminal experiments are certainly in their infancy. The authors evaluate the parallel development of minimally invasive thoracic surgery with regard to its counterpart in peritoneal laparoscopy to NOTES. Transesophageal interventions by both endosonographic and direct visualization are examined in the context of minimally invasive surgery and mediastinal NOTES. Techniques of viscerotomy creation, visualization, and closure are examined with particular emphasis on mediastinal structures. The state of current interventions is examined. Finally, current morbidity (including infectious complications) and survival outcomes are examined in those animals that have undergone transesophageal exploration.

THE CLINICS ARE NOW AVAILABLE ONLINE!

Access your subscription at:
www.theclinics.com

Preface

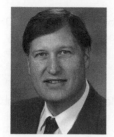

Herbert C. Wolfsen, MD
Guest Editor

In this issue of *Gastrointestinal Endoscopy Clinics of North America*, the authors have prepared articles that review all aspects of endosurgical technologies and devices that encompass endoluminal therapy for esophageal disease (Barrett's esophagus, squamous dysplasia, and carcinoma). Historically, one of the technologies that launched this area of clinical investigation is photodynamic therapy. Dr Seth A. Gross and I have reviewed the current status of photodynamic therapy and discussed where we believe it now fits into the spectrum of endotherapy options. Dr Frederike van Vilsteren and Dr Jacques Bergman have contributed a state-of-the art review of radiofrequency ablation, including careful practical descriptions of the endoscopic techniques developed at the Academic Medical Center in Amsterdam. Leaders in the development of cryotherapy, Dr Bruce Greenwald and his colleague, Dr Kevin D. Halsey, have written a comprehensive review of liquid nitrogen and carbon dioxide cryotherapy. An innovative pioneer who developed the devices and techniques for endoscopic resection and dissection, Dr Haruhiro Inoue has written an excellent review of his clinical experience. My clinical and research partners at the Mayo Clinic in Jacksonville, Florida, Dr Michael Wallace and Dr Timothy Woodward, have written comprehensive reviews of advanced endoscopic imaging and the use of natural orifice transluminal endoscopic surgery for esophageal disease. Drs Melina C. Vassiliou, Daniel von Renteln, and Richard I. Rothstein have contributed an excellent, state-of-the-art review of endoscopic therapy for gastroesophageal reflux disease, an area of esophageal therapy that has yet to capitalize on promising early work. Dr Bob Ganz has provided a thoughtful and intriguing glimpse into the endoscopic devices and technologies that are currently under development and will shape the future of clinical and research endoscopy. Finally, my colleague, Dr C. Daniel Smith, who is president of Society of American Gastrointestinal and Endoscopic Surgeons and chief of surgery at the Mayo Clinic in Jacksonville, Florida, has contributed a provocative comparative review of recent developments in surgical endoscopy, including minimally invasive esophagectomy.

Gastrointest Endoscopy Clin N Am 20 (2010) xi–xii
doi:10.1016/j.giec.2009.09.001
1052-5157/09/$ – see front matter © 2010 Elsevier Inc. All rights reserved.

As a long-time subscriber to *Gastrointestinal Endoscopy Clinics of North America*, it has been a wonderful experience to bring these manuscripts to publication. I hope all readers will find them equally useful and interesting.

Herbert C. Wolfsen, MD
Division of Gastroenterology and Hepatology
Mayo Clinic Florida
Jacksonville
FL, USA

Mayo Medical School
Rochester
MN, USA
E-mail address:
pdt@mayo.edu

Endoluminal Therapy for Esophageal Disease: An Introduction

Herbert C. Wolfsen, MD[a,b]

KEYWORDS

- Barrett esophagus • Argon plasma coagulation
- Cryotherapy • Endoscopic mucosal resection
- Multipolar electrocoagulation • Photodynamic therapy
- Radiofrequency ablation • Dysplasia

THE ENDOPREVENTION OF ESOPHAGEAL CANCER

This introductory article summarizes decades of research and clinical care from many dedicated gastrointestinal endoscopists. Pioneers such as Bergein Overholt, Charles Lightdale, and Kenneth Wang provided the scientific basis and clinical context for the development and use of esophageal endosonography and endoscopic resection and ablation. Not satisfied with diagnosing and staging esophageal cancer, they developed the endoscopic technology to detect and treat esophageal disease, to prevent the development of invasive cancer (endoprevention).[1] These developments paralleled my own career; one that began with Richard Kozarek at the Virginia Mason Clinic (Seattle), who had trained with Robert Sanowski, at the Maricopa County Veterans Administration Medical Center in Phoenix, Arizona. Dr Kozarek instilled in me an appreciation for gastrointestinal endoscopy, the importance of clinical research, and the need to support our professional societies, especially the American Society for Gastrointestinal Endoscopy (ASGE). My fellowship training with Kenneth Wang introduced me to cutting edge basic science and, clinical ablation research using photodynamic therapy, to understand disease mechanisms and investigate new treatments.

In 2003, the ASGE had established 3 new groups of members with specific interests, called SIGs (special interest groups). Soon thereafter, several endoscopic devices and technologies were developed for the treatment of Barrett disease. To create a forum to bring innovators and clinicians together, I asked more than 100 ASGE members to support a new SIG called Endoluminal Therapy for Esophageal Disease (ETED) in

a Division of Gastroenterology and Hepatology, Mayo Clinic Florida, 4500 San Pablo Road, Jacksonville, FL 32224, USA
b Mayo Medical School, Rochester, MN, USA
E-mail address: wolfsen.herbert@mayo.edu

Gastrointest Endoscopy Clin N Am 20 (2010) 1–10
doi:10.1016/j.giec.2009.07.006
1052-5157/09/$ – see front matter © 2010 Elsevier Inc. All rights reserved.

November, 2004. This broad and somewhat unwieldy term, suggested by Michael Kimmey and Michael Wallace at the 14th International Symposium on Endoscopic Ultrasonography (EUS 2004; Tokyo, Japan), was meant to include all gastrointestinal and surgical endoscopists, who used every type of resection or ablation technology and device in the treatment of esophageal diseases, malignant and premalignant.

The ETED SIG met for the first time on May 16, 2005, at Digestive Disease Week (DDW) in Chicago, Illinois, bringing together leading clinical researchers and industry innovators. This group, subsequently under the leadership of Bruce Greenwald and Drew Schembre, has continued to provide ASGE members with information and access to clinical experts, including sponsoring hands-on demonstration programs at DDW. Further, the ETED SIG has provided a platform to stimulate interaction and collaboration among ASGE members that are interested in new technologies for the diagnosis and treatment of Barrett disease, including the use of endoscopic therapy to prevent the development of esophageal cancer (endoprevention).

BARRETT ESOPHAGUS

Barrett esophagus (BE) develops as a result of chronic, pathologic reflux of gastro-duodenal contents into the esophagus. In North America, the diagnosis is considered based on the endoscopic finding of salmon-colored epithelium in the distal esophagus, followed by histologic confirmation of specialized intestinal columnar epithelium (specialized intestinal metaplasia [SIM]).[2,3] Barrett esophagus is estimated to be present in 1% to 2% of the US adult population,[3–6] with recent reports suggesting an increasing prevalence.[7,8] Rex and colleagues[7] reported a 6.8% prevalence in a general population of patients undergoing colonoscopy. In this study, as might be expected, the prevalence of SIM, was even higher (8.6%) among patients who reported gastroesophageal reflux disease (GERD) symptoms. In a Department of Veterans Affairs (VA) clinic study, Gerson and colleagues[8] reported a 25% prevalence of SIM in a predominantly white, male, non-GERD population (>50 years of age), undergoing sigmoidoscopy. The cause of this observed increase in the number of Barrett cases is unclear, but it may be related to the increase in the prevalence of patients reporting GERD, and increased awareness among gastroenterologists. The clinical importance of Barrett disease depends on the risks of progression to dysplasia and neoplasia in comparison with similar premalignant conditions.

RISK OF PROGRESSION TO DYSPLASIA AND ESOPHAGEAL ADENOCARCINOMA

The risk of a patient with nondysplastic Barrett esophagus progressing to esophageal adenocarcinoma has been reported to be 0.4% to 1% per patient per year,[9–11] a risk 30 to 125 times higher than the general population.[4,5,12] In 2005, according to the American Cancer Society, there were 14,520 new cases of esophageal cancer in the United States; most were cases of adenocarcinoma, and 13,570 deaths were associated with this disease.[13] This represents a 300% to 500% increase in US esophageal cancer incidence over the last 30 years.[6]

Sharma, and colleagues[9] reported that on the initial diagnosis of Barrett esophagus in 1376 patients (**Table 1**), a large number of patients had already developed low-grade dysplasia (LGD; 7.3%), high-grade dysplasia (HGD; 3.0%), or adenocarcinoma (6.0%). Subsequently, 618 of the nondysplastic SIM cases from this series underwent endoscopic surveillance for an average of 4 additional years. Over this time interval, a significant number of these previously nondysplastic patients progressed to LGD (16.1%), HGD (3.6%), or adenocarcinoma (2.0%) (**Table 2**). In this study, the annual risk of a patient with nondysplastic BE progressing to diagnosis of HGD or

Table 1 Incidence of dysplasia and cancer at initial diagnosis of BE		
Initial Diagnosis	Number	% of Cases
Intestinal metaplasia	1376	100
Low-grade dysplasia	101	7.3
High-grade dysplasia	42	3.0
Adenocarcinoma	91	6.7

adenocarcinoma, for which the standard of care is surgical esophagectomy, was 1.4% per patient (1 in 71 patients).

COLON ADENOMA/COLON AND RECTAL CARCINOMA VERSUS BE/ESOPHAGEAL ADENOCARCINOMA: A COMPARISON OF PREMALIGNANT CONDITIONS

According to the National Cancer Institute Surveillance, Epidemiology, and End Results data for 2005, the lifetime risk of developing colon and rectal carcinoma (CRC) is 5.7%, whereas that of esophageal cancer is 0.5%.[14] In 2005, there were 145,290 new cases of CRC in the United States, whereas there were 14,520 new cases of esophageal cancer. Although CRC has a much higher incidence than esophageal cancer (an approximately 10-fold difference), the age-adjusted death rate for CRC is 20.5 per 100,000 (population) versus 4.4 per 100,000 for esophageal cancer (less than a 5-fold difference). Furthermore, the CRC death rate for men of all races is 24.8 per 100,000 versus 7.7 per 100,000 for esophageal cancer (an approximately 3-fold difference). This difference in the incidence and death rate for CRC and esophageal cancer is due to the difference in 5-year survival for the 2 disease states: 64.1% for CRC versus 14.9% for esophageal cancer, with the latter being 1 of the lowest 5-year survival rates of any cancer diagnoses.

The risk of progression to CRC for a patient with polyps of the colon[15] and to esophageal adenocarcinoma for one with nondysplastic BE[9–11] are identical (0.5% per patient per year). The patient with BE may be found to progress to HGD (0.9% per patient per year), resulting in an aggregate risk (1.4% per patient per year) of developing a disease state for which the standard of care is esophagectomy.[9]

The surgical intervention for most CRC stages is segmental or hemicolectomy and for most esophageal cancer stages and HGD, is esophagectomy. The morbidity and mortality associated with removal of a segment of colon is low. However, esophagectomy carries a much higher risk for longer-term complications and death. Although mortality rates reported for esophagectomy in referral centers are typically 4% to 6%, several recent reports show that patients undergoing this operation in small,

Table 2 Progression of nondysplastic Barrett disease			
Diagnosis	Total	% Risk in 4 Years	% Risk Per Year
Total patients	618	NA	NA
Low-grade dysplasia	100	16.1	4.3
High-grade dysplasia	22	3.6	0.9
Adenocarcinoma	12	2.0	0.5

Abbreviation: NA, not applicable.

low-volume community hospitals incur a much higher mortality risk.[16,17] A recent US study examined 8657 cases that were treated between 1988 and 2000, and it evaluated the mortality associated with esophagectomy. A random sample of 20% of these cases showed that the overall in-hospital mortality rate was 11.3%, but it was lower in high-volume surgical centers, decreasing to 7.5%.[18] Additionally, several large studies have found that 30% to 50% of patients experienced at least 1 serious postoperative complication, such as pneumonia, myocardial infarction, heart failure, or wound infection, and that the average length of hospital stay was at least 2 weeks.[19] Late surgical complications, such as anastomotic strictures, are common, occurring in 10% to 56% of patients and require follow-up endoscopic dilation.[20] Respiratory function may remain depressed for 6 months after esophagectomy.[21] Removal of the gastroesophageal junction and relocation of the stomach remnant into the chest may be associated with severe, refractory, gastroesophageal reflux and long-term pulmonary complications; these procedures may even put a patient at risk of BE recurrence[22,23] and possible development of recurrent Barrett dysplasia or carcinoma.[23]

PREVENTION OF CRC AND HGD/ADENOCARCINOMA

After the advent of barium radiography of the colon, it was hypothesized that the development of CRC was preceded by malignant transformation of adenomatous polyps, and the subsequent development of the metaplasia-dysplasia-carcinoma sequence.[24] Other investigators, however, have cited the absence of residual adenomatous tissue in excised malignancies, and they suggest that colon cancers only rarely arise from adenomatous polyps.[25] Surveillance studies with matched cohorts, such as the National Polyp Study, found that patients undergoing endoscopic removal of adenomatous polyps were significantly less likely to develop colon carcinoma, a risk reduction of approximated 80% to 90%.[15] Subsequently, the use of screening colonoscopy and removal of colon polyps has been recognized as the most effective method for diagnosing and ultimately reducing the risk of developing CRC.[26] Therefore, the paradigm related to colon polyps and CRC prevention is: (1) screen candidate patients for colon polyps (ie, detect the precursor lesion for CRC); (2) remove the precursor lesion that has a 0.5% risk per patient per year of progression to CRC (ie, prevent progression to CRC).

Historically, the paradigm for BE and esophageal adenocarcinoma prevention has been strikingly different: (1) do not screen patients, but detect BE (precursor lesion for adenocarcinoma) incidentally, on endoscopy indicated for GERD symptoms; (2) once detected, do not remove the precursor lesion, even though the lesion incurs a 1.4% per patient per year risk of progressing to HGD or adenocarcinoma; (3) survey the nondysplastic BE patient every 3 years to detect progression to HGD or adenocarcinoma; (4) remove the esophagus when HGD or adenocarcinoma is detected.

RATIONALE FOR ENDOSCOPIC TREATMENT OF BARRETT DISEASE

Given the elevated risk, inherent in nondysplastic BE, of progression to HGD or adenocarcinoma, the conservative "watch and wait" approach being the standard of care for these patients needs explaining. There may be several reasons, such as (1) the limited ability to detect dysplasia in BE patients who undergo standard-resolution video or fiberoptic endoscopy, (2) the subsequent dependence on random biopsy protocols, and (3) the highly variable histopathology interpretations. Another explanation may be the absence of a technique for the safe, effective (complete), and reproducible removal of all SIM tissue in a patient.

There are multiple challenges inherent in achieving safe, effective, and reproducible removal of BE, and each of these factors must be considered when evaluating a technique for managing this disease: (1) access (the targeted portion of the esophagus is approximately 30 to 40 cm from the incisors); (2) irregular nature of the esophageal lumen (an uneven epithelial target); (3) mucous and gastric contents affecting delivery of the ablative energy; (4) esophageal motility; and (5) very tight margin between the ablation being "deep enough" (to the muscularis mucosae) and "too deep" (beyond the submucosa).

The ideal means to achieve safe, effective and reproducible ablation of BE requires a skilled endoscopist performing the interventional techniques to remove the Barrett epithelium entirely, without residual disease, especially subsquamous disease (buried glands). Endoscopic ablation methods should have a low rate of complication, such as stricture formation, bleeding, perforation, and must be well-tolerated by the patient. The endoluminal techniques that have been developed for removing BE include circumferential balloon-based radio-frequency ablation,[27–32] aminolevulinic acid and porfimer sodium photodynamic therapy,[33–49] endoscopic mucosal resection and submucosal dissection,[50–52] laser ablation,[4,53–59] argon plasma coagulation,[4,53,60–71] multipolar electrocoagulation,[4,53,72–76] and liquid nitrogen and carbon dioxide cryotherapy.[77–79]

However, these devices probably differ in their method of ablation, including in treatment depth. What depth of tissue ablation is required to effectively eliminate BE? In a study of resection specimens that were measured after tissue fixation and mounting, Ackroyd and colleagues[80] reported that the thickness of nondysplastic BE (500 ± 4 μm, range 390–590 μm) is similar to that of normal squamous epithelium (490 ± 3 μm, range 420–580 μm). These ex vivo data are useful information; if an ablation technique can be shown to repeatedly and uniformly penetrate at a minimum to the muscularis mucosae (approximately 700 μm) and at a maximum to the top of the submucosa (approximately 1000–1500 μm), then the Barrett epithelium can be reliably and safely removed. However, a recent study examined the use of endosonography to measure the esophageal wall thickness in BE patients with dysplasia and compared the results with a group of control patients.[81] In this study of 76 patients (most with LGD or HGD), the mean esophageal thickness was significantly greater for BE patients, compared with controls (3.36mm versus 2.4 mm, $P<.05$). There was also a trend toward increasing esophageal wall thickness with a greater degree of dysplasia, in BE patients, although these differences were not statistically significant. This raises important questions regarding differences among BE patients, the methods used to measure mucosal disease, and how these differences may alter treatment outcomes. These variability factors include thickness of Barrett esophageal wall layers, blood flow, and mucosal oxygenation; these factors are important for developing dosimetry systems to monitor the effect of esophageal ablation therapy of all types, for delivering optimal results and for avoiding complications, such as incomplete ablation, stricture, or perforation.[82] Some of this ex vivo disease-depth information was subsequently used in the development of radiofrequency energy ablation (RFA). The use of RFA in a prospective multi-center randomized controlled trial of patients with Barrett LGD and HGD was recently reported in the *New England Journal of Medicine*.[83] At a follow-up of 12 months, among patients with LGD, complete eradication of dysplasia occurred in 90.5% in the ablation group compared with 22.7% in the control group ($P<.001$). Among patients with HGD, complete eradication occurred in 81.0% of those in the ablation group compared with 19.0% of those in the control group ($P<.001$). RFA-treated patients had less disease progression (36% versus 16.3%, $P = .03$) and fewer cancers (1.2% versus 9.3%, $P = .045$). Complications in RFA-treated patients were limited to bleeding in 1 patient and stricture in 5 patients (6.0%). These early results represent important progress toward the goal of an ideal form of endoscopic therapy for Barrett disease. Yet, a small number of patients did experience dysplasia progression, including cancer despite the use of RFA; questions remain about the durability of these results and whether they can be achieved outside of elite endoscopy centers. How to select patients for treatment (risk stratification) and whether nondysplastic BE patients should be treated remain to be investigated in long-term controlled studies.[84] Despite these limitations, studies such as these move us steadily closer to ideal endoscopic treatment modalities for the safe, effective, reproducible, stable, and durable treatment of Barrett disease, to prevent the development of dysplasia or carcinoma.

REFERENCES

1. Wolfsen HC. Endoprevention of esophageal cancer: endoscopic ablation of Barrett's metaplasia and dysplasia. Expert Rev Med Devices 2005;2(6):713–23.
2. Spechler SJ. Clinical practice. Barrett's Esophagus. N Engl J Med 2002;346(11): 836–42.
3. Peters JH, Hagen JA, DeMeester SR. Barrett's esophagus. J Gastrointest Surg 2004;8(1):1–17.
4. Eisen GM. Ablation therapy for Barrett's esophagus. Gastrointest Endosc 2003; 58(5):760–9.
5. Reid BJ. Barrett's esophagus and esophageal adenocarcinoma. Gastroenterol Clin North Am 1991;20(4):817–34.
6. Shaheen N, Ransohoff DF. Gastroesophageal reflux, Barrett esophagus, and esophageal cancer: scientific review. JAMA 2002;287(15):1972–81.
7. Rex DK, Cummings OW, Shaw M, et al. Screening for Barrett's esophagus in colonoscopy patients with and without heartburn. Gastroenterology 2003;125(6): 1670–7.
8. Gerson LB, Shetler K, Triadafilopoulos G. Prevalence of Barrett's esophagus in asymptomatic individuals. Gastroenterology 2002;123(2):461–7.
9. Sharma D, Reker D, Falk G, et al. Progression of Barrett's esophagus to high-grade dysplasia and cancer: preliminary results of the BEST trial [abstract]. Gastroenterology 2001;120:16.
10. O'Connor JB, Falk GW, Richter JE. The incidence of adenocarcinoma and dysplasia in Barrett's esophagus: report on the Cleveland Clinic Barrett's Esophagus Registry. Am J Gastroenterol 1999;94(8):2037–42.
11. Drewitz DJ, Sampliner RE, Garewal HS. The incidence of adenocarcinoma in Barrett's esophagus: a prospective study of 170 patients followed 4.8 years. Am J Gastroenterol 1997;92(2):212–5.
12. Provenzale D, Kemp JA, Arora S, et al. A guide for surveillance of patients with Barrett's esophagus. Am J Gastroenterol 1994;89(5):670–80.
13. American Cancer Society. Cancer facts & figures 2005. Atlanta (GA): The Society; 2005.
14. Ries LAG, Eisner MP, Kosary CL, et al. In: SEER cancer statistics review, 1975–2002, vol. 2005. Bethesda: National Cancer Institute; 2005.
15. Winawer SJ, Zauber AG, Ho MN, et al. Prevention of colorectal cancer by colonoscopic polypectomy. The National Polyp Study Workgroup. N Engl J Med 1993; 329(27):1977–81.
16. Urbach DR, Baxter NN. Does it matter what a hospital is "high volume" for? Specificity of hospital volume-outcome associations for surgical procedures: analysis of administrative data. BMJ 2004;328(7442):737–40.

17. Bartels H, Stein HJ, Siewert JR. Risk analysis in esophageal surgery. Recent Results Cancer Res 2000;155:89–96.
18. Dimick JB, Wainess RM, Upchurch GR Jr, et al. National trends in outcomes for esophageal resection. Ann Thorac Surg 2005;79(1):212–6 [discussion: 17–8].
19. Lerut TE, van Lanschot JJ. Chronic symptoms after subtotal or partial oesophagectomy: diagnosis and treatment. Best Pract Res Clin Gastroenterol 2004; 18(5):901–15.
20. Orringer MB, Marshall B, Iannettoni MD. Eliminating the cervical esophagogastric anastomotic leak with a side-to-side stapled anastomosis. J Thorac Cardiovasc Surg 2000;119(2):277–88.
21. Ikeguchi M, Maeta M, Kaibara N. Respiratory function after esophagectomy for patients with esophageal cancer. Hepatogastroenterology 2002;49(47): 1284–6.
22. Shibuya S, Fukudo S, Shineha R, et al. High incidence of reflux esophagitis observed by routine endoscopic examination after gastric pull-up esophagectomy. World J Surg 2003;27(5):580–3.
23. Wolfsen HC, Hemminger LL, DeVault KR. Recurrent Barrett's esophagus and adenocarcinoma after esophagectomy. BMC Gastroenterol 2004;4(1):18.
24. Bond JH. Interference with the adenoma-carcinoma sequence. Eur J Cancer 1995;31A(7–8):1115–7.
25. Castleman B, Krickstein HI. Do adenomatous polyps of the colon become malignant? Nord Hyg Tidskr 1962;267:469–75.
26. Rex DK, Johnson DA, Lieberman DA, et al. Colorectal cancer prevention 2000: screening recommendations of the American College of Gastroenterology. American College of Gastroenterology. Am J Gastroenterol 2000;95(4):868–77.
27. Ganz RA, Utley DS, Stern RA, et al. Complete ablation of esophageal epithelium with a balloon-based bipolar electrode: a phased evaluation in the porcine and in the human esophagus. Gastrointest Endosc 2004;60(6):1002–10.
28. Sharma D, Overholt B, Wang K, et al. A randomized multi-center evaluation of ablation of nondysplastic short segment Barrett's esophagus using BARRX bipolar balloon device: extended follow-up of the Ablation of Intestinal Metaplasia (AIM-I) Trial [abstract]. Gastrointest Endosc 2005;61(5):239.
29. Sharma VK, McLaughlin R, Dean P, et al. Successful ablation of Barrett's esophagus with low-grade dysplasia using BARRX bipolar balloon device: Preliminary results of the Ablation of Intestinal Metaplasia with LGD (AIM-LGD) Trial [abstract]. Gastrointest Endosc 2005;61(5):143.
30. Dunkin BJ, Martinez J, Bejarano PA, et al. Thin layer ablation of human esophageal epithelium using a bipolar radiofrequency balloon device. Surg Endosc 2006;20(1):125–30.
31. Smith CD, Dunkin BJ, Bejarano PA, et al. Thin-layer ablation of intestinal metaplasia with high-grade dysplasia in esophagectomy patients using a bipolar radiofrequency balloon device (BARRX System) [abstract]. Gastroenterology 2005;128(4):809.
32. Fleischer DE, Sharma VK, Reymunde A, et al. A prospective multi-center evaluation of ablation of non-dysplastic Barrett's esophagus using the BARRX bipolar balloon device [abstract]. Ablation of Intestinal Metaplasia Trial (AIM-II). Gastroenterology 2005;128(4):236.
33. Overholt BF, Lightdale CJ, Wang KK, et al. Photodynamic therapy with porfimer sodium for ablation of high-grade dysplasia in Barrett's esophagus: international, partially blinded, randomized phase III trial. Gastrointest Endosc 2005;62(4): 488–98.

34. Wang K. Photodynamic therapy made simple. Clin Perspect Gastroenterol 2001;90–100.
35. Webber J, Herman M, Kessel D, et al. Current concepts in gastrointestinal photodynamic therapy. Ann Surg 1999;230(1):12–23.
36. Kubba AK. Role of photodynamic therapy in the management of gastrointestinal cancer. Digestion 1999;60(1):1–10.
37. Prosst RL, Wolfsen HC, Gahlen J. Photodynamic therapy for esophageal diseases: a clinical update. Endoscopy 2003;35(12):1059–68.
38. DeVault KR, Ward EM, Wolfsen HC, et al. Barrett's esophagus (BE) is common in older patients undergoing screening colonoscopy regardless of gastroesophageal reflux (GER) symptoms [abstract]. Gastrointest Endosc 2004;59:AB111.
39. Wolfsen HC, Hemminger LL. Photodynamic therapy for dysplastic Barrett's esophagus and mucosal adenocarcinoma [abstract]. Gastrointest Endosc 2004;59(5):AB251.
40. Wang KK, Wong Kee Song LM, Buttar NS, et al. Barrett's esophagus after photodynamic therapy: risk of cancer development during long term follow up [abstract]. Gastroenterology 2004;126(Suppl 2):A50.
41. Wang KK. Current status of photodynamic therapy of Barrett's esophagus. Gastrointest Endosc 1999;49(3 Pt 2):S20–3.
42. Wolfsen HC, Woodward TA, Raimondo M. Photodynamic therapy for dysplastic Barrett esophagus and early esophageal adenocarcinoma. Mayo Clin Proc 2002;77(11):1176–81.
43. Wang KK, Kim JY. Photodynamic therapy in Barrett's esophagus. Gastrointest Endosc Clin N Am 2003;13(3):483–9, vii.
44. Wolfsen HC. Photodynamic therapy for mucosal esophageal adenocarcinoma and dysplastic Barrett's esophagus. Dig Dis 2002;20(1):5–17.
45. Overholt BF, Panjehpour M, Haydek JM. Photodynamic therapy for Barrett's esophagus: follow-up in 100 patients. Gastrointest Endosc 1999;49(1):1–7.
46. Malhi-Chowla N, Wolfsen HC, DeVault KR. Esophageal dysmotility in patients undergoing photodynamic therapy. Mayo Clin Proc 2001;76(10):987–9.
47. Ban S, Mino M, Nishioka NS, et al. Histopathologic aspects of photodynamic therapy for dysplasia and early adenocarcinoma arising in Barrett's esophagus. Am J Surg Pathol 2004;28(11):1466–73.
48. Vij R, Triadafilopoulos G, Owens DK, et al. Cost-effectiveness of photodynamic therapy for high-grade dysplasia in Barrett's esophagus. Gastrointest Endosc 2004;60(5):739–56.
49. Nijhawan PK, Wang KK. Endoscopic mucosal resection for lesions with endoscopic features suggestive of malignancy and high-grade dysplasia within Barrett's esophagus. Gastrointest Endosc 2000;52(3):328–32.
50. Soetikno RM, Gotoda T, Nakanishi Y, et al. Endoscopic mucosal resection. Gastrointest Endosc 2003;57(4):567–79.
51. Conio M, Cameron AJ, Chak A, et al. Endoscopic treatment of high-grade dysplasia and early cancer in Barrett's oesophagus. Lancet Oncol 2005;6(5):311–21.
52. May A, Gossner L, Behrens A, et al. A prospective randomized trial of two different endoscopic resection techniques for early stage cancer of the esophagus. Gastrointest Endosc 2003;58(2):167–75.
53. Haag S, Nandurkar S, Talley NJ. Regression of Barrett's esophagus: the role of acid suppression, surgery, and ablative methods. Gastrointest Endosc 1999;50(2):229–40.

54. Gossner L, May A, Stolte M, et al. KTP laser destruction of dysplasia and early cancer in columnar-lined Barrett's esophagus. Gastrointest Endosc 1999;49(1): 8–12.
55. Salo JA, Salminen JT, Kiviluoto TA, et al. Treatment of Barrett's esophagus by endoscopic laser ablation and antireflux surgery. Ann Surg 1998;227(1):40–4.
56. Bonavina L, Ceriani C, Carazzone A, et al. Endoscopic laser ablation of nondysplastic Barrett's epithelium: is it worthwhile? J Gastrointest Surg 1999;3(2):194–9.
57. Barham CP, Jones RL, Biddlestone LR, et al. Photothermal laser ablation of Barrett's oesophagus: endoscopic and histological evidence of squamous re-epithelialisation. Gut 1997;41(3):281–4.
58. Luman W, Lessels AM, Palmer KR. Failure of Nd-YAG photocoagulation therapy as treatment for Barrett's oesophagus–a pilot study. Eur J Gastroenterol Hepatol 1996;8(7):619–30.
59. Weston AP, Sharma P. Neodymium:yttrium-aluminum garnet contact laser ablation of Barrett's high grade dysplasia and early adenocarcinoma. Am J Gastroenterol 2002;97(12):2998–3006.
60. Ginsberg GG, Barkun AN, Bosco JJ, et al. The argon plasma coagulator: February 2002. Gastrointest Endosc 2002;55(7):807–10.
61. Tigges H, Fuchs KH, Maroske J, et al. Combination of endoscopic argon plasma coagulation and antireflux surgery for treatment of Barrett's esophagus. J Gastrointest Surg 2001;5(3):251–9.
62. Basu KK, Pick B, Bale R, et al. Efficacy and one year follow up of argon plasma coagulation therapy for ablation of Barrett's oesophagus: factors determining persistence and recurrence of Barrett's epithelium. Gut 2002;51(6):776–80.
63. Morino M, Rebecchi F, Giaccone C, et al. Endoscopic ablation of Barrett's esophagus using argon plasma coagulation (APC) following surgical laparoscopic fundoplication. Surg Endosc 2003;17(4):539–42.
64. Schulz H, Miehlke S, Antos D, et al. Ablation of Barrett's epithelium by endoscopic argon plasma coagulation in combination with high-dose omeprazole. Gastrointest Endosc 2000;51(6):659–63.
65. Byrne JP, Armstrong GR, Attwood SE. Restoration of the normal squamous lining in Barrett's esophagus by argon beam plasma coagulation. Am J Gastroenterol 1998;93(10):1810–5.
66. Mork H, Barth T, Kreipe HH, et al. Reconstitution of squamous epithelium in Barrett's oesophagus with endoscopic argon plasma coagulation: a prospective study. Scand J Gastroenterol 1998;33(11):1130–4.
67. Van Laethem JL, Cremer M, Peny MO, et al. Eradication of Barrett's mucosa with argon plasma coagulation and acid suppression: immediate and mid term results. Gut 1998;43(6):747–51.
68. Pereira-Lima JC, Busnello JV, Saul C, et al. High power setting argon plasma coagulation for the eradication of Barrett's esophagus. Am J Gastroenterol 2000;95(7):1661–8.
69. Grade AJ, Shah IA, Medlin SM, et al. The efficacy and safety of argon plasma coagulation therapy in Barrett's esophagus. Gastrointest Endosc 1999;50(1): 18–22.
70. Van Laethem JL, Jagodzinski R, Peny MO, et al. Argon plasma coagulation in the treatment of Barrett's high-grade dysplasia and in situ adenocarcinoma. Endoscopy 2001;33(3):257–61.
71. Dulai GS, Jensen DM, Cortina G, et al. Randomized trial of argon plasma coagulation vs. multipolar electrocoagulation for ablation of Barrett's esophagus. Gastrointest Endosc 2005;61(2):232–40.

72. Montes CG, Brandalise NA, Deliza R, et al. Antireflux surgery followed by bipolar electrocoagulation in the treatment of Barrett's esophagus. Gastrointest Endosc 1999;50(2):173–7.
73. Sharma P, Sampliner RE, Camargo E. Normalization of esophageal pH with high-dose proton pump inhibitor therapy does not result in regression of Barrett's esophagus. Am J Gastroenterol 1997;92(4):582–5.
74. Kovacs BJ, Chen YK, Lewis TD, et al. Successful reversal of Barrett's esophagus with multipolar electrocoagulation despite inadequate acid suppression. Gastrointest Endosc 1999;49(5):547–53.
75. Sampliner RE, Faigel D, Fennerty MB, et al. Effective and safe endoscopic reversal of nondysplastic Barrett's esophagus with thermal electrocoagulation combined with high-dose acid inhibition: a multicenter study. Gastrointest Endosc 2001;53(6):554–8.
76. Fennerty MB, Corless CL, Sheppard B, et al. Pathological documentation of complete elimination of Barrett's metaplasia following endoscopic multipolar electrocoagulation therapy. Gut 2001;49(1):142–4.
77. Johnston CM, Schoenfeld LP, Mysore JV, et al. Endoscopic spray cryotherapy: a new technique for mucosal ablation in the esophagus. Gastrointest Endosc 1999;50(1):86–92.
78. Rodgers BM, McDonald AP, Talbert JL, et al. Morphologic and functional effects of esophageal cryotherapy. J Thorac Cardiovasc Surg 1979;77(4):543–9.
79. Grana L, Ablin RJ, Goldman S, et al. Freezing of the esophagus: histological changes and immunological response. Int Surg 1981;66(4):295–301.
80. Ackroyd R, Brown NJ, Stephenson TJ, et al. Ablation treatment for Barrett oesophagus: what depth of tissue destruction is needed? J Clin Pathol 1999; 52(7):509–12.
81. Gill K, Nawaz I, Crook J, et al. Variation in Barrett's Esophageal Wall Thickness: Is it associated with histology and length? Gastrointest Endosc 2008;67(5):200 [abstract].
82. Gill KR, Wolfsen HC, Preyer NW, et al. Pilot study on light dosimetry variables for photodynamic therapy of Barrett's esophagus with high-grade dysplasia. Clin Cancer Res 2009;15(5):1830–6.
83. Shaheen NJ, Sharma P, Overholt BF, et al. Radiofrequency ablation in Barrett's esophagus with dysplasia. N Engl J Med 2009;360(22):2277–88.
84. Bergman JJ. Radiofrequency ablation–great for some or justified for many? N Engl J Med 2009;360(22):2353–5.

Endoscopic Imaging for the Detection of Esophageal Dysplasia and Carcinoma

Muhammad W. Shahid, MD, Michael B. Wallace, MD, MPH*

KEYWORDS

- Barrett's • Endoscopy • Chromoendoscopy • NBI
- Auto-fluorescence • Confocal • Spectroscopy • OCT

WHITE-LIGHT ENDOSCOPIC IMAGING

Standard videoendoscopy magnifies an image approximately 5 to 10 times and gives an image resolution of 100,000 to 300,000 pixels. A pixel is a photosensitive element that generates an electrical charge in proportion to light exposure and then generates an analog signal that is digitalized by a computer video processor. Image resolution (ie, the ability to discriminate between 2 adjacent points) achieved with a standard video endoscope is not sufficient, as the focal distance of these endoscopes is only 1 to 9 cm. This distance restricts the ability of standard white-light endoscopes to detect dysplasia and early carcinoma with precision, as any lesion beyond the range of this focal distance will not appear clear. Hence, quadratic mucosal biopsies are required to make the diagnosis. However, biopsy sampling is associated with certain issues such as increased cost, more time required, more sampling errors, and high interobserver variability in histopathological diagnosis.[1] Techniques are needed that can easily differentiate normal from abnormal mucosa, to guide and, if possible, eliminate the need for biopsies. High-resolution endoscopes (HRE) are a newer class of endoscope that better detect microscopic mucosal abnormalities because of their ability to produce images with higher magnification (of up to 100 times) and increased spatial resolution of 600,000 to 1 million pixels. HRE are equipped with movable lenses, resulting in variable focal distance. These qualities allow more detailed examination of the mucosal, glandular, and vascular structures at a range of less than 3 mm.

Division of Gastroenterology and Hepatology, Mayo Clinic, 4500 San Pablo Road, Jacksonville, FL 32224, USA
* Corresponding author.
E-mail address: wallace.michael@mayo.edu (M.B. Wallace).

Gastrointest Endoscopy Clin N Am 20 (2010) 11–24
doi:10.1016/j.giec.2009.08.006
1052-5157/09/$ – see front matter © 2010 Elsevier Inc. All rights reserved.

CHROMOENDOSCOPY

Chromoendoscopy involves endoscopic examination of gastrointestinal mucosa after applying a dye solution to the surface, which enhances the appearance of otherwise nonperceivable mucosal changes. This technique guides the endoscopist to take target biopsies only from the suspicious areas. Different dye solutions are used including Lugol iodine solution, methylene blue (MB), indigo carmine, crystal violet, and acetic acid. Lugol solution consists of a 0.5% to 3.0% aqueous solution of potassium iodide, and iodine and is taken up by glycogen-containing cells. It is more useful for detecting dysplasia in patients with increased risk of squamous cell carcinoma (ie, with a history of smoking, alcoholism, and lye ingestion). On the other hand, MB, indigo carmine, and acetic acid are more useful in the detection of glandular abnormalities, as seen in adenocarcinoma. After staining with these agents, different mucosal patterns become visible during videoendoscopy. Various studies have been done to classify and detect dysplasia and early carcinoma based on these patterns. Guelrud and colleagues[2] used acetic acid, a mucolytic agent, to stain the esophageal mucosa, and observed 4 pit patterns (round, reticular, villous, and ridged). Villous and ridged patterns were found to be associated with intestinal metaplasia. Sharma and colleagues[3] studied the mucosal changes in 80 patients with Barrett esophagus (BE) after application of indigo carmine, and observed 3 mucosal patterns: ridged/villous, circular, and irregular/distorted. The irregular/distorted pattern was found to be associated with Barrett high-grade dysplasia (HGD) or superficial adenocarcinoma in 6 patients. In the same study, the presence of the ridged or villous pattern had 97% sensitivity, 76% specificity, and 92% positive predictive value (PPV) for prediction of intestinal metaplasia. However, in subsequent studies, these results could not be reproduced and no detection benefit for either Barrett metaplasia or dysplasia could be established with chromoendoscopy.[4,5] Other studies using acetic acid and crystal violet stain also produced variable results.[6,7,8] The probable reasons for these conflicting observations could be differences in technique, operator experience, and a patient population with a prevalence of BE.[9,10] This was further substantiated in a blinded European study in which 4 expert gastrointestinal endoscopists analyzed magnification chromoendoscopy images of BE, using acetic acid or MB. The interobserver agreement was poor ($\kappa = 0.40$) for all parameters studied, including the mucosal patterns, MB positive staining, and the presence of specialized intestinal metaplasia (SIM).[11]

Ngamruengphong and colleagues[12] performed a meta-analysis of 9 studies published in PubMed for assessment of the diagnostic yield of techniques of chromoendoscopy compared with conventional 4-quadrant random biopsy (RB) in detection of SIM and dysplasia in patients with BE. A total of 450 patients with BE were reported in 9 studies included in the meta-analysis. Data on the yield of both modalities were extracted and analyzed to estimate weighted incremental yield (IY) and 95% confidence intervals (CIs) of MB chromoendoscopy with target biopsies over RB protocol using the Cochrane Q χ^2 test. There was no significant IY with MB over RB for detection of SIM (IY 4%; 6 studies, n = 251), dysplasia (IY 9%; 9 studies, n = 450), and HGD or early cancer (EC) (IY 5%; 8 studies, n = 405). This meta-analysis shows that the technique of MB chromoendoscopy only has a comparable yield with white-light endoscopy using RBs for the detection of SIM and dysplasia during endoscopic evaluation of patients with BE.[12]

Ormeci and colleagues[13] compared conventional endoscopy with chromoendoscopy in 109 patients using MB. The sensitivity of chromoendoscopy for Barrett epithelium was superior to that of conventional endoscopy (87% compared with

66%; $P<.05$): However, there was no statistical difference between the 2 methods in the diagnosis of esophageal carcinoma ($P>.05$). They concluded that chromoendoscopy is useful for delineating Barrett epithelium and for indicating the correct location for securing biopsies when dysplasia or early esophageal cancer is suspected.

MB is a vital dye with intracellular binding characteristics, and safety issues have been raised regarding possible DNA damage associated with white-light illumination.[14] These concerns, along with high cost, long procedure time, and unreliable detection of mucosal abnormalities, have impaired the widespread application of vital dye staining chromoendoscopy techniques in clinical practice.[11]

NARROW-BAND IMAGING

The working principal of narrow-band imaging (NBI) is based on the use of light filters which reduce red and green light and preserve the amount of blue light that illuminates the tissue. The resultant blue-green excitation light with narrow bandwidth has limited optical scattering and shallow penetration depth. It improves the imaging of mucosal and glandular changes and efficiently visualizes abnormal vascular patterns. As blue light is readily taken up by hemoglobin, NBI successfully detects the increased density of abnormal microvessels that is associated with dysplasia and carcinoma.[15]

This technology was first introduced by Gono and colleagues[16] in 1999 as a combined effort of the Japanese National Cancer Center Hospital East and a team of bio-optical physicists from Olympus Corporation (Tokyo, Japan). There are 2 versions of the NBI system. One version is called the Evis Exera II system, which is predominately used in North America. It is equipped with several diminutive band-pass color filters that allow green light of 530 to 550 nm bandwidth and blue light of 390 to 445 nm bandwidth to pass through and activate each pixel on a trichromatic charge-coupled device (CCD). The other system is the Lucera system, which uses a monochromatic CCD system and is used predominantly in Japan and Europe. Both systems allow switching between high-resolution white-light and NBI modes using a switch on the handle of endoscope. Although they have slight technical differences, the systems are functionally similar.

NBI has several advantages over vital dye chromoendoscopy in terms of applicability, cost, time, tidiness, and precision. It is widely available commercially and has already received regulatory approval. It is one of the most extensively studied advanced endoscopic imaging techniques for the detection of esophageal dysplasia and superficial carcinoma.

The mucosal and vascular patterns seen in BE have been the basis of many single-center studies (**Fig. 1**). Kara and colleagues[17] studied these patterns in BE patients and observed the association of regular mucosal and vascular patterns with intestinal metaplasia, whereas irregular mucosa and abnormal blood vessels were present in Barrett HGD. In another study, Kara and colleagues[18,19] compared HRE with indigo carmine chromoendoscopy or NBI in 14 patients with Barrett HGD. The aim of the study was to compare and correlate the findings with the combinations of these techniques for the detection of Barrett HGD or superficial carcinoma. Eleven patients with HGD (79%) were detected with HRE alone, whereas NBI found HGD in 12 patients (86%). Indigo carmine was able to detect HGD in 13 patients (93%), whereas HGD (7%) was found in 1 patient using RB, which could not be detected with any imaging modality. NBI found an additional 4 HGD lesions in 3 of these 12 patients. White-light resolution endoscopy detected all cases of HGD, showing better efficacy for primary detection than NBI. However, NBI was more useful for detailed inspection of suspicious lesions. As a historical comparison, a previous study performed by this group

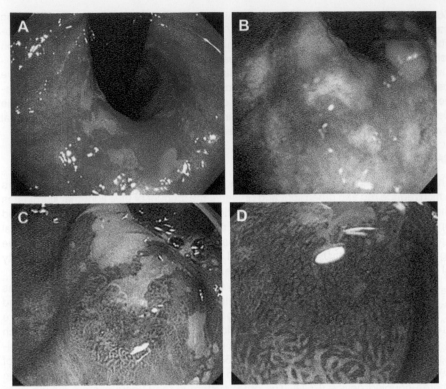

Fig. 1. A BE lesion with HGIN detected with AFI. (*A*) During inspection with white light, this area was not judged as suspicious. (*B*) The area around the small squamous island in the middle of the image showed a blue-violet autofluorescence imaging color. (*C, D*) With NBI, irregular and disrupted mucosal patterns were found. The histopathology confirmed the presence of HGIN. (*From* Curvers WL, Singh R, Song LM, et al. Endoscopic tri-modal imaging for detection of early neoplasia in Barrett's oesophagus: a multi-centre feasibility study using high-resolution endoscopy, autofluorescence imaging and narrow band imaging incorporated in one endoscopy system. Gut 2008;57(2):167–72; with permission.)

detected HGD in 62% of patients using targeted standard resolution endoscopy (SRE) biopsies, and in 85% of patients with SRE-targeted plus random quadrantic biopsies.[18,19]

Anagnostopoulos[20] studied mucosal and vascular features of Barrett disease in 50 patients with 344 lesions using high-resolution magnification endoscopy and NBI. The sensitivity, specificity, positive and negative predictive values of regular mucosal, and vascular patterns for intestinal metaplasia were 100%, 79%, 94%, and 100% respectively, whereas sensitivity, specificity, positive and negative predictive values for HGD in these patients were 90%, 100%, 99%, and 100%, respectively.[20]

Curvers and colleagues[21] performed a blinded study involving 14 patients with 22 suspicious lesions, including 8 lesions of HGD, 1 lesion with low-grade dysplasia, 1 lesion indefinite for dysplasia, and 12 areas of nondysplastic Barrett disease. They performed high-resolution endoscopy with vital dye staining techniques, using acetic acid and indigo carmine and NBI. In a blinded fashion, 7 community and 5 expert gastrointestinal endoscopists evaluated standard images from these lesions for any association of glandular and vascular patterns with dysplasia. The detection rate for dysplasia or neoplasia, with high-resolution white-light endoscopy, was 86% overall (90% for experts and 84% for nonexperts). The addition of vital dye staining or NBI did not improve the diagnostic yield. By contrast, Herrero and colleagues[22] evaluated a simplified NBI classification of mucosal morphology to assess inter- and intraobserver agreement and the correlation with histology. Two hundred NBI images were evaluated twice by 4 endoscopists experienced in NBI and 4 inexperienced endoscopists at 2 referral centers. Endoscopists assessed each image for quality, suspicion for dysplasia, and regularity of mucosal and vascular patterns. Overall interobserver agreement was seen to be moderate (κ 0.42–0.44), whereas overall intraobserver agreement was moderate to substantial (κ 0.60–0.62). However, endoscopists in this study correctly identified 71% of the images containing HGD/EC and 68% of nondysplastic images were correctly identified as not suspicious. There were no significant differences in agreement between expert and inexpert endoscopists, suggesting a short "learning curve." This low rate of identification of HGD/EC (71%) contrasts with the previous studies, cited previously, and Singh's[23] prospective single-center study involving 21 patients with BE, comparing the imaging characteristics between high-resolution magnification white-light endoscopy and NBI with histology. Mucosal patterns (pit pattern and microvascular morphology) were evaluated for their image quality on a visual analog scale of 1 to 10 by 5 expert endoscopists who then predicted mucosal changes based on pit and microvascular patterns. NBI was superior to white-light endoscopy in the prediction of histology in BE, as the overall pit and microvasculature quality was significantly higher ($P<.001$). Furthermore, NBI was also observed to be superior to white-light endoscopy for prediction of dysplasia ($\chi^2 = 10.3$, $P<.05$). The overall κ agreement among the 5 endoscopists was 0.59 and 0.31 ($P<.001$) showing good reproducibility.[23] Although these "off-line" studies that review images from procedures have generally confirmed the usefulness of NBI for the diagnosis of Barrett disease and the detection of dysplasia, the low rate of identification of HGD/EC (71%) in the Herrero[22] study raises questions regarding the ability of NBI to replace the use of RB protocols for surveillance endoscopy in BE patients.

In a prospective, blinded, tandem study, our group at Mayo Clinic compared SRE and HRE-NBI in 65 patients with BE. With HRE-NBI, dysplasia was detected in 37 patients (57%), whereas SRE with targeted plus RBs detected dysplasia in 28 patients (43%), which was statistically significant ($P<.001$). NBI also found higher grades of dysplasia in 12 patients (18%), compared with no cases of SRE, with targeted plus RBs, detecting a high grade of histology (0%; $P<.001$). This study also showed greater efficiency of HRE-NBI, as fewer NBI-directed biopsies (mean 4.7 biopsies per case; $P<.001$) were needed to detect dysplasia in significantly more patients with BE, compared with SRE with targeted plus RBs (mean 8.5 biopsies per case). Sharma and colleagues[24] presented the results of a prospective, multicenter, randomized crossover trial of HRE with quadrantic biopsy protocol compared with HRE with NBI-targeted biopsies for dysplasia detection in 116 patients undergoing screening or surveillance for BE. Overall, there was no significant difference between the 2 modalities in the primary aim of detecting intestinal metaplasia (HRE 85%, NBI 86%, $P = .61$). However, NBI detected HGD and cancer (23%) more often compared with HRE, even though the proportion of patients with neoplasia as not statistically different between the groups (HRE 29%, NBI 34%, $P = .22$). HRE detected 1 of 3 cancers and 7 of 10 HGD patients, whereas NBI detected all 3 cancers and 8 of 10 HGD patients. NBI also detected significantly more lesions with HGD/cancer than HRE (17 vs 10, $P = .03$) and more overall lesions with any degree of dysplasia compared with HRE (71 vs 55, $P = .0002$). NBI also required fewer biopsies per procedure (3.7 vs 8.0, $P<.0001$). This study showed that, although the overall rate of intestinal metaplasia detection was similar between HRE and NBI, NBI achieved this with fewer biopsies per procedure and had significantly better detection rates for neoplastic lesions.[24] These clinical studies demonstrate the importance of HRE in combination with NBI for the surveillance evaluation of BE patients.[25–27] Further, NBI is the most rigorously studied method of "virtual chromoendoscopy," with controlled studies suggesting that the use of NBI improves the accuracy and efficiency of dysplasia detection in BE patients.

CONFOCAL LASER ENDOMICROSCOPY AND ENDOCYTOSCOPY

A major milestone in endoscopic-based enhanced imaging technology is the development of confocal laser endomicroscopy (CLE). This promising new technology enables real-time, in vivo microscopic imaging of esophageal mucosa. The basic principal of confocal endomicroscopy involves stimulation of mucosal cells with blue laser excitation light after tissues have been exposed to topical or intravenous fluorescent contrast agents, acriflavine, or fluorescein, respectively. The reflected light is captured and transmitted through a pinhole to eliminate out-of-focus light. It is then transferred by numerous optic fibers to a laser scanning unit (LSU), which then generates black and white cross-sectional histologic images of the mucosa. Two systems have been developed based on this technology. The endoscope-integrated system (eCLE) has been developed by OptiScan with Pentax, Japan, and consists of an endoscope with integrated confocal laser system. It permits magnification beyond 1000 times with cellular and subcellular resolution of epithelial, glandular, and vascular architecture to a depth of 250 μm (the level of the lamina propria). An extra advantage of eCLE lies in the stability achieved during acquisition of the images with the help of a suction device. However, a major limitation is the requirement for a dedicated confocal endoscope made by a single endoscope manufacturer. Thus, the decision to use confocal imaging in a particular case requires the purchase of specific endoscopes, and the use of those endoscopes in each case, which makes the use of this system cumbersome in clinical practice. Initial studies using this system have reported high accuracy (85%–94%) for the detection of HGD in BE.[28,29]

The other CLE system has been developed by Mauna Kea Technologies, France, and is based on a miniature laser probe-based CLE (pCLE). This probe is thin enough to be passed through the accessory channel of any endoscope, making it more practical and easy to use in clinical practice. This system also provides resolution of more than 1000 times the normal for real-time endoscopic microscopy at varying depths from 50 to 120 μm.[30] It features postprocedure image reconstruction for video mosaicing, the combination of dynamic single-frame images into a static, mosaic image over a broad field, without reduction in image resolution.[31] Both systems use the application of intravenous fluorescein or topical contrast agent such as acriflavine or cresyl violet. Within 30 seconds of its injection, fluorescein is distributed through the capillaries to the mucosal tissue and is taken up by epithelial and other cells. Subcellular compartments, such as cytoplasm, containing the fluorescein appear bright, whereas cellular structures that do not take up fluorescein, such as nuclei, appear dark. Vessels that have fluorescein flowing in the plasma also appear as bright cords. Dysplastic cells fail to take up fluorescein, and appear dark. Thus, the cellular and architectural details of the tissues become visible. These characteristic confocal features are used to differentiate neoplastic, preneoplastic, and benign lesions of the esophagus (**Fig. 2**).

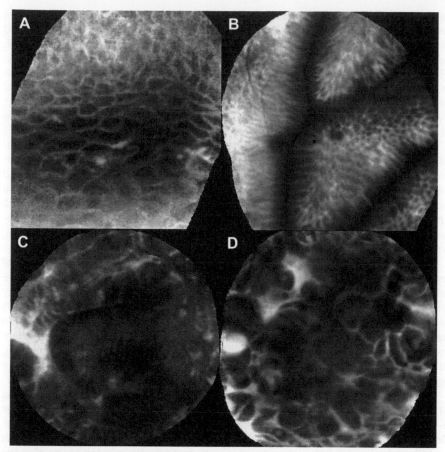

Fig. 2. pCLE imaging. (A) Normal squamous epithelium in esophagus. (B) BE without dysplasia. (C) High-grade dysplasia. (D) Carcinoma.

Wallace and colleagues[32] evaluated the accuracy and interobserver agreement of 9 international endoscopists in pCLE in patients with BE-associated dysplasia. Forty BE sites were imaged with pCLE using high-definition probe ultra-high definition (UHD), and corresponding biopsies were obtained at 3 different centers from the United States and Europe. The pCLE video sequences were randomized and divided into a teaching set and a validation set, each consisting of 20 videos. Each investigator was provided with histopathologic diagnosis during viewing of a standardized teaching set. The 20 videos of the validation set were evaluated and assessed for histology. The overall accuracy of pCLE for the diagnosis of HGD of the 9 experts was 90.5%, sensitivity 88%, and specificity 94% (range 75%–100%). Of the 9 endoscopists, the 3 most experienced endomicroscopists had an overall accuracy of 97%, sensitivity 94%, and specificity 100%. The interobserver agreement for all 9 experts was good (intraclass correlation coefficient 0.72; 95% CI 0.57–0.85).

Dunbar and colleagues[33] designed a prospective, double-blind, randomized, cross-over study to evaluate the difference in diagnostic yields of eCLE with targeted biopsy and standard endoscopy (SE) with a 4-quadrant RB in endoscopically unapparent,

BE-associated neoplasia. Thirty nine BE patients completed the study, 16 of whom were suspected to have HGD, and 23 underwent surveillance of BE. CLE with targeted biopsy significantly improves the diagnostic yield for endoscopically unapparent BE neoplasia (33.7%) compared with a SE with a random-biopsy protocol (17%) (P<.01).The CLE with targeted biopsy also resulted in a 59% reduction in the number of biopsies needed per patient compared with SE-RB (9.8 biopsies vs 23.8 biopsies) and allows some patients without neoplasia to completely forgo mucosal biopsy. Two-thirds of patients in the surveillance group did not need any mucosal biopsies at all during CLE examination.

Kiesslich and colleagues[28] evaluated the ability of CLE for detection of BE and associated neoplasia during ongoing high-resolution endoscopy in 63 patients. Endomicroscopy distinguished between different types of epithelial cells and detected cellular and vascular changes in Barrett epithelium. BE and associated neoplasia could be predicted with a sensitivity of 98.1% and 92.9% and a specificity of 94.1% and 98.4%, respectively (accuracy, 96.8% and 97.4%). The mean κ value for interobserver agreement for the prediction of histopathological diagnosis was high (0.843), whereas the intraobserver agreement showed a high mean κ value of 0.892.

Pohl and colleagues[34] designed and conducted a prospective 2-center, 2-phase trial using pCLE during standard high-resolution endoscopy: phase I to establish pCLE criteria for detection of Barrett neoplasia and phase II to test these criteria on 296 biopsy sites in 38 consecutive patients with BE. Miniprobe confocal laser microscopy (CLM) showed a high negative predictive value for the diagnosis of endoscopically invisible neoplasia in BE. In a per biopsy analysis, sensitivity and specificity for 2 independent investigators were 75.0% and 88.8%, and 75.0% and 91.0%, respectively, translating at best into a PPV of 44.4% and a negative predictive value of 98.8%. Interobserver agreement was good (κ 0.6); sensitivity, however, has still to be improved.

Endocytoscopy involves imaging of cellular and subcellular structures in vivo using high-magnification endoscopes or small-caliber magnification probes (outer diameter 3.4 mm) that are passed through the working channel of any therapeutic endoscope. Before microscopic examination, tissues are stained with a dye or contrast agent such as MB, and magnification probes are placed in contact with mucosa to visualize the cellular and nuclear details. The endocytoscopy does not require the use of fluorescent agent and laser light for excitation of fluorophores as applied in CLE. This technology enables magnifications of up to 450 or 1125 times, essentially allowing the identification of single cells and nuclei in a sampling area that is less than 0.5 mm in diameter. Pohl and colleagues[35] performed an ex vivo study of 166 biopsy sites from 16 BE patients using endocytoscopy. The endocytoscopy images were obtained after application of MB and were analyzed in a blinded study by a gastroenterologist and a pathologist. At most, 23% of images with lower magnification and 41% of higher magnification images could be interpreted to identify characteristics of dysplasia and neoplasia. The sensitivity and specificity were 43% and 85%, respectively, at high magnification, and 50% and 67%, respectively, at low magnification for diagnosing dysplasia or cancer in BE. Interobserver agreement was less than fair (κ <0–0.45), with positive and negative predictive values for HGD or carcinoma of 0.29 and 0.87, respectively, for 450× magnification, and 0.44 and 0.83, respectively, for 1125× magnification.

Eberl and colleagues[36] studied 76 patients using endocytoscopy with MB. Twenty five of these patients had unspecified esophageal lesions. The endocytoscopic images were evaluated in a blinded study by 2 pathologists. At high magnification, the sensitivity and specificity were found to be 91% and 100%, respectively, whereas at lower magnification, they were 71% and 100% for both pathologists.

The real-time use of endocytoscopy in vivo is likely to be limited by image stabilization problems, with motion artifact and image distortion. The requirement of a pathologist for the interpretation of the endocytoscopic images may also prevent more widespread use of this technology.

AUTOFLUORESCENCE IMAGING

Autofluorescence imaging (AFI) is a technique that differentiates tissue types (normal vs abnormal) based on their differences in fluorescence emission. The exposure of the tissue to light of a shorter wavelength leads to emission of a longer wavelength of light due to the excitation of endogenous biologic substances (fluorophores). In the gastrointestinal tract, AFI can detect differences in autofluorescence as a result of subtle changes in the concentration of these specific chemicals occurring as a result of neoplastic proliferation. The molecules that lead to tissue autofluorescence include NADH, collagen, flavin, elastin, aromatic amino acids, and porphyrins. AFI uses blue light illumination to excite the tissue, producing a low-intensity autofluorescence that is detected through highly sensitive CCDs, along with reflectance imaging detected through nonintensified CCD.[37] The malignant transformation of tissue leads to emission of longer wavelengths of light (shifting from green toward the red end of the spectrum).[38,39] Earlier studies in which AFI was used with fiber-optic scopes were unable to show any differences when compared with white-light endoscopy because of poor white-light images.[20,40,41] However, in an uncontrolled study of 60 patients with BE, Kara and colleagues[42] detected HGD in 22 patients. In 6 of these patients, white-light endoscopy was unable to detect dysplastic lesions, but AFI did find those lesions. Therefore, AFI detected a significant number of patients with HGD, increasing the target detection rate from 63% to 91%. However, AFI testing was associated with a 51% false-positive rate, as the biopsies of 41 of 81 suspicious areas by AFI did not have dysplasia, which shows its poor specificity.

The international multicenter study by Curvers and colleagues[43] showed that the addition of AFI to HRE did increase the detection of the number of lesions and the number of patients with early neoplasia in patients with BE. In this study, the false-positive rate of AFI was reduced by detailed inspection with NBI. This randomized crossover trial of 130 patients compared the diagnostic accuracy of surveillance with AFI-guided plus 4-quadrant biopsies with the conventional approach. The investigators suggested that the AFI-guided approach improved the diagnostic yield for neoplasia in comparison with the conventional approach using 4-quadrant biopsies. However, it was concluded that, because of decreased sensitivity, AFI alone was not suitable for replacing the standard 4-quadrant biopsy protocol.[44]

SPECTROSCOPY

Light-scattering spectroscopy is a novel technique that uses the variation in scattered light across a full spectrum to obtain information about the size and number of nuclei of a cellular layer.[38] This technique may detect mucosal abnormalities in real time, using molecular and microstructural information in light-tissue interactions.[45] This technique has been reported to be promising, with high accuracy in detecting dysplasia in BE.[46,47] Epithelial cell nuclei are the primary targets of reflected light that is singly scattered before it is collected by the probe. This imaging modality may be an important breakthrough technology, although more data and controlled studies are required for validation. Different spectroscopic techniques can be used to obtain information about the histologic characterization of gut tissue. Reflectance spectroscopy quantitatively measures the color and intensity of reflected light after tissue illumination, to differentiate normal from abnormal mucosa. Hemoglobin is the primary molecule that absorbs light and, on the basis of tissue oxygenation, provides information about angiogenesis and dysplasia.

Raman spectroscopy detects scattered light that has been slightly changed in wavelength (inelastic scattering), as a result of energy transfer between light and mucosa molecules. These shifts correspond to specific vibrations of molecular bonds. During this process, some of the energy is transferred to the molecules so the light emitted back from the tissue is reduced in energy and has a longer wavelength. Raman spectra form multiple peaks and bands that produce detailed tissue character-ization. However, due to weak Raman signals, near-infrared light is typically used for excitation and sophisticated detection instruments, and signal processing computers are required. Raman spectroscopy has recently been applied to the detection of Barrett associated dysplasia, with promising results.[48,49]

Panjehpour and colleagues[50] used laser-induced autofluorescence spectroscopy to differentiate normal esophageal mucosa from dysplastic and malignant tissue, with high accuracy. Mayinger and colleagues[51] used a filtered ultraviolet-blue light source and showed that there were specific differences in the emitted autofluores-cence spectra of esophageal carcinoma with normal mucosa. In another study, Bourg-Heckly and colleagues[52] reported a sensitivity and specificity of 86% and 95%, respectively, in the identification of HGD in BE and EC using light spectroscopy. However, they were not able to distinguish nondysplastic Barrett mucosa from squa-mous mucosa by this technique. Stael von Holstein and colleagues[27,54] and Brand and colleagues[53] used the exogenous fluorophore photosensitizer porfimer sodium and photosensitizer 5-aminolevulinic acid (5-ALA) to distinguish normal and dysplastic tissue in an in vitro study of esophagectomy specimens. Ortner and colleagues[55] were able to enhance the features of dysplastic BE by combing time-resolved fluores-cence spectroscopy and topical application of 5-ALA. Trimodal spectroscopy is a novel technique, and few data are available. In their study, Georgakoudi and colleagues[46] used trimodal spectroscopy and showed sensitivity and specificity to distinguish HGD from non-HGD in BE to be 100%, and dysplastic versus nondysplas-tic BE to be 93% and 100% respectively.

OPTICAL COHERENCE TOMOGRAPHY

Optical coherence tomography (OCT) was first used in 1997. Initial time domain OCT systems had limited image speed and sensitivity.[56] Subsequently, the development of Fourier domain OCT has provided better imaging speed and sensitivity, and has greater potential to perform three-dimensional imaging in real time. OCT is similar to endoscopic ultrasound in acquiring tissue images, but it uses light instead of sound. OCT uses short coherence-length broad-band light for micrometer-sized cross-sectional imaging of the gut mucosa. However, because of limited development of the image-detection devices (scanning probes), clinical application is cumbersome and not yet commercially available.[57,58]

CONCLUSIONS AND THE FUTURE OF IMAGING FOR BE

This article outlines recent advancements in enhanced esophageal imaging for detec-tion of dysplasia and EC. Some of these modalities are still being reviewed for practical application, clinical usefulness, and regulatory approval. Of the currently available enhancement modalities, high-resolution white-light endoscopy (HRE), NBI, and chromoendoscopy have shown clinical benefit, practical and easy applicability, and widespread commercial availability of the equipment. These are widely used in routine clinical practice, especially in academic referral endoscopy centers, and have been approved by the Food and Drug Administration (FDA) in the United States. Fujinon intelligent color enhancement (FICE, Fujinon), spectroscopy, OCT, and iScan (Pentax) have also passed regulatory approval and are currently under investigation for their clinical usefulness. CLE imaging is rapidly emerging as a useful tool in practice and is undergoing further study. Other ongoing validation studies are focused on the use of the endoscopic trimodal imaging system that combines the wide-field detection capabilities of HRE with AFI and NBI. Regulatory approval for the use of the combination systems has already been granted in Europe, and approval in America is expected in the near future.

However, unresolved issues that need to be addressed involving some of these technologies include commercial availability, securing reimbursement for the required additional time and imaging equipment, and clarifying the medical-legal issues associated with image interpretation and data storage. In the long term, the future of imaging for detection of dysplasia and early carcinoma is likely to be associated with the development of molecular targeting probes (such as monoclonal antibodies) that have been conjugated to dyes or nanoparticles. These sensitive and specific devices will serve as diagnostic molecular beacons, and as delivery systems for therapeutic agents.[45]

REFERENCES

1. Spechler SJ, Goyal RK. The columnar-lined esophagus, intestinal metaplasia, and Norman Barrett. Gastroenterology 1996;110(2):614–21.
2. Guelrud M, Herrera I, Essenfeld H, et al. Enhanced magnification endoscopy: a new technique to identify specialized intestinal metaplasia in Barrett's esophagus. Gastrointest Endosc 2001;53(6):559–65.
3. Sharma P, Weston AP, Topalovski M, et al. Magnification chromoendoscopy for the detection of intestinal metaplasia and dysplasia in Barrett's oesophagus. Gut 2003;52(1):24–7.
4. Lim CH, Rotimi O, Dexter SP, et al. Randomized crossover study that used methylene blue or random 4-quadrant biopsy for the diagnosis of dysplasia in Barrett's esophagus. Gastrointest Endosc 2006;64(2):195–9.
5. Wo JM, Ray MB, Mayfield-Stokes S, et al. Comparison of methylene blue-directed biopsies and conventional biopsies in the detection of intestinal metaplasia and dysplasia in Barrett's esophagus: a preliminary study. Gastrointest Endosc 2001;54(3):294–301.
6. Amano Y, Kushiyama Y, Ishihara S, et al. Crystal violet chromoendoscopy with mucosal pit pattern diagnosis is useful for surveillance of short-segment Barrett's esophagus. Am J Gastroenterol 2005;100(1):21–6.
7. Ferguson DD, DeVault KR, Krishna M, et al. Enhanced magnification-directed biopsies do not increase the detection of intestinal metaplasia in patients with GERD. Am J Gastroenterol 2006;101(7):1611–6.
8. Hoffman A, Kiesslich R, Bender A, et al. Acetic acid-guided biopsies after magnifying endoscopy compared with random biopsies in the detection of Barrett's esophagus: a prospective randomized trial with crossover design. Gastrointest Endosc 2006;64(1):1–8.
9. Armstrong D. Review article: towards consistency in the endoscopic diagnosis of Barrett's oesophagus and columnar metaplasia. Aliment Pharmacol Ther 2004; 20(Suppl 5):40–7 [discussion: 61–2].

10. Canto MI. Chromoendoscopy and magnifying endoscopy for Barrett's esophagus. Clin Gastroenterol Hepatol 2005;3(7 Suppl 1):S12–5.
11. Canto MI, Kalloo A. Chromoendoscopy for Barrett's esophagus in the twenty-first century: to stain or not to stain? Gastrointest Endosc 2006;64(2):200–5.
12. Ngamruengphong S, Sharma V, Das A. Diagnostic yield of methylene blue chromoendoscopy for detecting specialized intestinal metaplasia and dysplasia in Barrett's esophagus: a meta-analysis. Gastrointest Endosc 2009;69(6):1021–8.
13. Ormeci N, Savas B, Coban S, et al. The usefulness of chromoendoscopy with methylene blue in Barrett's metaplasia and early esophageal carcinoma. Surg Endosc 2008;22(3):693–700.
14. Olliver JR, Wild CP, Sahay P, et al. Chromoendoscopy with methylene blue and associated DNA damage in Barrett's oesophagus. Lancet 2003;362(9381):373–4.
15. Sharma P, Bansal A, Mathur S, et al. The utility of a novel narrow band imaging endoscopy system in patients with Barrett's esophagus. Gastrointest Endosc 2006;64(2):167–75.
16. Gono K, Obi T, Yamaguchi M, et al. Appearance of enhanced tissue features in narrow-band endoscopic imaging. J Biomed Opt 2004;9(3):568–77.
17. Kara MA, Ennahachi M, Fockens P, et al. Detection and classification of the mucosal and vascular patterns (mucosal morphology) in Barrett's esophagus by using narrow band imaging. Gastrointest Endosc 2006;64(2):155–66.
18. Kara MA, Peters FP, Rosmolen WD, et al. High-resolution endoscopy plus chromoendoscopy or narrow-band imaging in Barrett's esophagus: a prospective randomized crossover study. Endoscopy 2005;37(10):929–36.
19. Kara MA, Smits ME, Rosmolen WD, et al. A randomized crossover study comparing light-induced fluorescence endoscopy with standard videoendoscopy for the detection of early neoplasia in Barrett's esophagus. Gastrointest Endosc 2005;61(6):671–8.
20. Anagnostopoulos GK, Yao K, Kaye P, et al. Novel endoscopic observation in Barrett's oesophagus using high resolution magnification endoscopy and narrow band imaging. Aliment Pharmacol Ther 2007;26(3):501–7.
21. Curvers WL, Singh R, Wong Kee Song LM, et al. Endoscopic tri-modal imaging for detection of early neoplasia in Barrett's oesophagus; a multi-centre feasibility study using high-resolution endoscopy, autofluorescence imaging and narrow band imaging incorporated in one endoscopy system. Gut 2007;39(Suppl I):A1.
22. Herrero LA, Curvers WL, Bansal A, et al. Zooming in on Barrett oesophagus using narrow-band imaging: an international observer agreement study. Eur J Gastroenterol Hepatol 2009;21(9):1068–75.
23. Singh R, Karageorgiou H, Owen V, et al. Comparison of high-resolution magnification narrow-band imaging and white-light endoscopy in the prediction of histology in Barrett's oesophagus. Scand J Gastroenterol 2009;44(1):85–92.
24. Sharma P, Bansal A, Hawes R, et al. Detection of metaplasia (IM) and neoplasia in patients with Barrett's esophagus (BE) using high-definition white light endoscopy (HD-WLE) versus narrow band imaging (NBI): a prospective, multi-center, randomized, crossover trial. Gastrointest Endosc 2009;69(5):AB135.
25. Sharma P, Bansal A. Toward better imaging of Barrett's esophagus–see more, biopsy less!. Gastrointest Endosc 2006;64(2):188–92.
26. Gheorghe C. Narrow-band imaging endoscopy for diagnosis of malignant and premalignant gastrointestinal lesions. J Gastrointestin Liver Dis 2006;15(1):77–82.
27. Wolfsen HC, Crook JE, Krishna M, et al. Prospective, controlled tandem endoscopy study of narrow band imaging for dysplasia detection in Barrett's esophagus. Gastroenterology 2008;135(1):24–31.

28. Kiesslich R, Gossner L, Goetz M, et al. In vivo histology of Barrett's esophagus and associated neoplasia by confocal laser endomicroscopy. Clin Gastroenterol Hepatol 2006;4(8):979–87.
29. Polglase AL, McLaren WJ, Skinner SA, et al. A fluorescence confocal endomicroscope for in vivo microscopy of the upper- and the lower-GI tract. Gastrointest Endosc 2005;62(5):686–95.
30. Meining A, Saur D, Bajbouj M, et al. In vivo histopathology for detection of gastrointestinal neoplasia with a portable, confocal miniprobe: an examiner blinded analysis. Clin Gastroenterol Hepatol 2007;5(11):1261–7.
31. Becker V, Vercauteren T, von Weyhern CH, et al. High-resolution miniprobe-based confocal microscopy in combination with video mosaicing (with video). Gastrointest Endosc 2007;66(5):1001–7.
32. Wallace MB, et al. Accuracy and inter-observer agreement of experts for probe-based confocal laser endomicroscopy detection of dysplasia in Barrett's esophagus. Gastrointest Endosc 2009;69(5):AB351.
33. Dunbar KB, Okolo P 3rd, Montgomery E, et al. Confocal laser endomicroscopy in Barrett's esophagus and endoscopically inapparent Barrett's neoplasia: a prospective, randomized, double-blind, controlled, crossover trial. Gastrointest Endosc 2009; June 24 [Epub ahead of print].
34. Pohl H, Rosch T, Vieth M, et al. Miniprobe confocal laser microscopy for the detection of invisible neoplasia in patients with Barrett's oesophagus. Gut 2008; 57(12):1648–53.
35. Pohl H, Koch M, Khalifa A, et al. Evaluation of endocytoscopy in the surveillance of patients with Barrett's esophagus. Endoscopy 2007;39(6):492–6.
36. Eberl T, Jechart G, Probst A, et al. Can an endocytoscope system (ECS) predict histology in neoplastic lesions? Endoscopy 2007;39(6):497–501.
37. Kara M, DaCosta RS, Wilson BC, et al. Autofluorescence-based detection of early neoplasia in patients with Barrett's esophagus. Dig Dis 2004;22(2): 134–41.
38. Buchner AM, Wallace MB. Future expectations in digestive endoscopy: competition with other novel imaging techniques. Best Pract Res Clin Gastroenterol 2008;22(5):971–87.
39. Reddymasu SC, Sharma P. Advances in endoscopic imaging of the esophagus. Gastroenterol Clin North Am 2008;37(4):763–74, vii.
40. Egger K, Werner M, Meining A, et al. Biopsy surveillance is still necessary in patients with Barrett's oesophagus despite new endoscopic imaging techniques. Gut 2003;52(1):18–23.
41. Niepsuj K, Niepsuj G, Cebula W, et al. Autofluorescence endoscopy for detection of high-grade dysplasia in short-segment Barrett's esophagus. Gastrointest Endosc 2003;58(5):715–9.
42. Kara MA, Peters FP, Ten Kate FJ, et al. Endoscopic video autofluorescence imaging may improve the detection of early neoplasia in patients with Barrett's esophagus. Gastrointest Endosc 2005;61(6):679–85.
43. Curvers WL, Singh R, Song LM, et al. Endoscopic tri-modal imaging for detection of early neoplasia in Barrett's oesophagus: a multi-centre feasibility study using high-resolution endoscopy, autofluorescence imaging and narrow band imaging incorporated in one endoscopy system. Gut 2008;57(2): 167–72.
44. Borovicka J, Fischer J, Neuweiler J, et al. Autofluorescence endoscopy in surveillance of Barrett's esophagus: a multicenter randomized trial on diagnostic efficacy. Endoscopy 2006;38(9):867–72.

45. Wilson BC. Detection and treatment of dysplasia in Barrett's esophagus: a pivotal challenge in translating biophotonics from bench to bedside. J Biomed Opt 2007; 12(5):051401.
46. Georgakoudi I, Jacobson BC, Van Dam J, et al. Fluorescence, reflectance, and light-scattering spectroscopy for evaluating dysplasia in patients with Barrett's esophagus. Gastroenterology 2001;120(7):1620–9.
47. Wallace MB, Perelman LT, Backman V, et al. Endoscopic detection of dysplasia in patients with Barrett's esophagus using light-scattering spectroscopy. Gastroenterology 2000;119(3):677–82.
48. Kendall C, Stone N, Shepherd N, et al. Raman spectroscopy, a potential tool for the objective identification and classification of neoplasia in Barrett's oesophagus. J Pathol 2003;200(5):602–9.
49. Wong Kee Song LM. Optical spectroscopy for the detection of dysplasia in Barrett's esophagus. Clin Gastroenterol Hepatol 2005;3(7 Suppl 1):S2–7.
50. Panjehpour M, Overholt BF, Schmidhammer JL, et al. Spectroscopic diagnosis of esophageal cancer: new classification model, improved measurement system. Gastrointest Endosc 1995;41(6):577–81.
51. Mayinger B, Horner P, Jordan M, et al. Endoscopic fluorescence spectroscopy in the upper GI tract for the detection of GI cancer: initial experience. Am J Gastroenterol 2001;96(9):2616–21.
52. Bourg-Heckly G, Blais J, Padilla JJ, et al. Endoscopic ultraviolet-induced autofluorescence spectroscopy of the esophagus: tissue characterization and potential for early cancer diagnosis. Endoscopy 2000;32(10):756–65.
53. Brand S, Wang TD, Schomacker KT, et al. Detection of high-grade dysplasia in Barrett's esophagus by spectroscopy measurement of 5-aminolevulinic acid-induced protoporphyrin IX fluorescence. Gastrointest Endosc 2002;56(4): 479–87.
54. von Holstein CS, Nilsson AM, Andersson-Engels S, et al. Detection of adenocarcinoma in Barrett's oesophagus by means of laser induced fluorescence. Gut 1996;39(5):711–6.
55. Ortner MA, Ebert B, Hein E, et al. Time gated fluorescence spectroscopy in Barrett's oesophagus. Gut 2003;52(1):28–33.
56. Bouma BE, Tearney GJ, Compton CC, et al. High-resolution imaging of the human esophagus and stomach in vivo using optical coherence tomography. Gastrointest Endosc 2000;51(4 Pt 1):467–74.
57. Evans JA, Poneros JM, Bouma BE, et al. Optical coherence tomography to identify intramucosal carcinoma and high-grade dysplasia in Barrett's esophagus. Clin Gastroenterol Hepatol 2006;4(1):38–43.
58. Qi X, Sivak MV, Isenberg G, et al. Computer-aided diagnosis of dysplasia in Barrett's esophagus using endoscopic optical coherence tomography. J Biomed Opt 2006;11(4):044010.

Endoscopic Mucosal Resection and Endoscopic Submucosal Dissection for Esophageal Dysplasia and Carcinoma

Haruhiro Inoue, MD, PhD, FASGE*, Hitomi Minami, MD, Makoto Kaga, MD,
Yoshitaka Sato, MD, Shin-ei Kudo, MD, PhD

KEYWORDS

- Endoscopic mucosal resection
- Endoscopic submucosal dissection
- Esophageal dysplasia • Carcinoma

Advanced cancer in the esophagus is a serious and fatal disease that invades locally to deeper layers of the esophageal wall with significant risk of nodal metastasis and invasion of adjacent organs. One reliable method of avoiding this is to detect lesions at an early stage of esophageal cancer and then to resect them locally.[1–6] A major advantage of endoscopic local resection is to recover a specimen for histopathologic analysis, which allows one to make a clinical decision for further therapy. Once cancer invades into the submucosal layer and/or permeates into the lymphatic vessel, additional surgery or chemoradiotherapy becomes necessary if there is to be any hope for a complete cure from the disease. This is because there is 0% risk of lymph node metastasis for cancers limited to the mucosa, but there is a 16% to 22% risk for cancers that extend into the submucosa.[7] Tumor biology may also be important because well-differentiated carcinomas usually involve the mucosa only (93%). By comparison, only 74% and 23% of moderately and poorly differentiated carcinomas, respectively, are confined to the submucosa.[8] Indication for endoscopic local resection of esophageal neoplasia is a superficial lesion of the esophagus with no risk of lymph node metastasis. From histologic analysis of the surgically resected specimen, mucosal cancer (high-grade intramucosal neoplasia) generally has an extremely low risk of lymph node metastasis. Endoscopic mucosal resection (EMR) and endoscopic

Digestive Disease Center, Showa University, Northern Yokohama Hospital, Chigasaki Chuo 35-1, Tsuzuki-ku, Yokohama 224-8503, Japan
* Corresponding author.
E-mail address: haruinoue777@yahoo.co.jp (H. Inoue).

Gastrointest Endoscopy Clin N Am 20 (2010) 25–34
doi:10.1016/j.giec.2009.08.005
1052-5157/09/$ – see front matter © 2010 Elsevier Inc. All rights reserved.

submucosal dissection (ESD) have already been established as techniques of endoscopic local resection. EMR includes strip-off biopsy, double-channel techniques, cap technique, EMR using a ligating device, and so on. ESD is a newly developed technique in which submucosal dissection is carried out using an electro-cautery knife to acquire a single-piece specimen.

In this article, the EMR-cap technique[9] and ESD using a triangle-tip knife[10] are intro-duced, both of which were devised by the authors. The cap technique is a fast and easy procedure to perform, and it is mostly applied to a relatively small lesion (around 1 cm). The triangle-tip (TT) knife is applied to a larger lesion for a one-piece resection.

PRINCIPLES OF ENDOSCOPIC LOCAL RESECTION

The esophageal wall basically consists of 2 major components: the mucosal layer and the muscle layer. Embryologically, the mucosa develops from the endoderm, and the muscle layer is derived from the mesoderm. These 2 components are attached to each other by the loose connective tissue of the submucosa and can be easily sepa-rated by an external force. For this reason, it is possible to resect only the mucosa, leaving the muscle layer intact. However, the esophageal wall is just 4 mm thick, and therefore special management is necessary to create a technically safe working space between the mucosa and muscle layer. Saline injection into the submucosal layer is the easiest and most cost-effective technique for separating the 2 layers. Lift-ing of the mucosal surface is always observed after correct submucosal injection of the saline. After a sufficient volume of saline has been injected, the mucosa, including the target lesion, can be safely captured with the cap or can be dissected with an electrocautery knife.

EMR USING A CAP-FITTED ENDOSCOPE

The steps involved in EMR using a cap-fitted endoscope (EMR-C) are described in the following sections. "Cap" here refers to an attachment on the distal tip of the forward-viewing endoscope, and it is made of a transparent plastic material.

Preparation

In preparation for the EMR-C procedure, a cap is attached to the tip of the forward-viewing endoscope and is fixed tightly with an adhesive tape. For the initial session of EMR in the esophagus, an obliquely cut large-capacity cap with a rim (Olympus MAJ297, Tokyo, Japan; **Fig. 1**A) is most commonly used by fixing it onto the tip of the standard size endoscope. By using this large cap, a large sample can be obtained. For trimming a residual lesion, if necessary, a straight-cut medium-size cap with a rim (Olympus MH595, see **Fig. 1**B) is appropriate. All of the items needed for the EMR-C procedure are present in an EMR kit (Olympus).

Markings

The mucosal surface that surrounds the margin of the lesion is carefully marked by the tip of the snare wire. Markings are positioned 2 mm away from the actual lesion margin. This is important because the appearance of the lesions and its margins may become dramatically distorted and difficult to recognize after submucosal injec-tion (see later discussion). The image enhancement produced by chromoendoscopy disappears within a couple of minutes. On the other hand, marking by electrocautery lasts longer, which helps easy recognition of lesion margin, especially for a flat lesion.

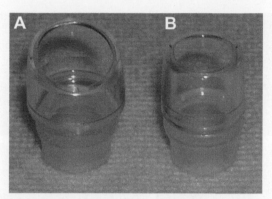

Fig. 1. Distal attachment "cap" for EMR. (*A*) Large, oblique cap with rim; outer diameter, 16.5 mm. This large cap is applied to a first capture during the EMR-C procedure. Around 2 cm of mucosa can be resected en bloc. (*B*) Medium, straight cap with rim; outer diameter, 13.5 mm. This cap is used to trim the lesion. Approximately 1 cm of mucosa can be resected en bloc.

Injection

A diluted epinephrine/saline solution (0.5 mL of 0.1% epinephrine solution plus 100 mL of normal saline) is injected into the submucosa with an injection needle (23 gauge; tip length, 4 mm). Puncturing the target mucosa at a sharp angle is the most important key to avoiding transmural penetration of the needle tip (**Fig. 2**B). The total volume of injected saline depends on the size of the lesion, but it is necessary to inject enough saline to lift up the whole lesion. Usually, more than 20 mL epinephrine/saline is injected. Normal mucosa that is distal to the lesion is first punctured. When saline is accurately injected into the submucosal layer, lifting or bulging of the mucosa is always observed in any part of esophageal wall (see **Fig. 2**).

Prelooping of the Snare Wire

A specially designed small-diameter snare (outer diameter,1.8 mm; Olympus SD-7P) is essential for the prelooping process. The snare wire is fixed along the rim of the cap. To create prelooping conditions, moderate suction is first applied to the normal mucosa to seal the outlet of the cap, and the snare wire that passes through the endoscope instrument channel is then opened. The opened snare wire is fixed along the rim of the cap, and the snare's outer sheath sticks up to the rim of the cap (see **Fig. 2**C). This completes the prelooping process for the snare wire.

Suction of the Target Mucosa

The prelooping position is maintained as the endoscope is brought near the target mucosa. The target mucosa, including the lesion, is fully sucked inside the cap (see **Fig. 2**D, E) and is strangulated by simple closing of the prelooped snare wire. At this moment, the strangulated mucosa looks like a snared polypoid lesion (see **Fig. 2**F, G).

Resection

The pseudopolyp of strangulated mucosa is cut using blended-current electrocautery. The resected specimen can easily be taken out by keeping it inside the cap without using any grasping forceps. The smooth surface of the proper muscle layer is observed at the bottom of the artificial ulcer (see **Fig. 2**H).

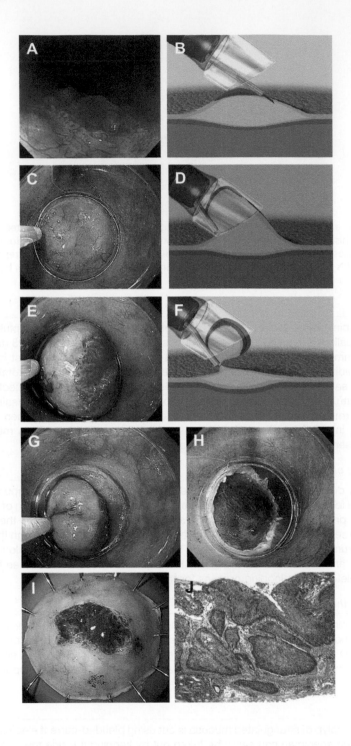

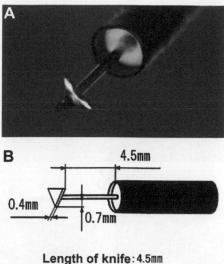

Length of knife: 4.5mm
Thickness of tip: 0.4mm
Length of tip: 0.7mm

Fig. 3. Image of triangle-tip knife (*A*). Triple angles help to capture and dissect the tissue in any direction. A drawing of triangle knife (*B*).

Additional Resection

If additional resection is necessary to remove the residual lesion completely, all of the processes, including saline injection, should be repeated step by step. The injected saline usually infiltrates and disappears within a few minutes at the initial injection site, so that it no longer acts as a cushion between the mucosa and muscle layer.

◀

Fig. 2. (*A*) Endoscopic view. Lesion with nodular surface was easily identified with regular endoscopy. Surface irregularity suggests that invasion of this lesion may be submucosal. (*B*) Schematic drawing of submucosal injection. The cap is premounted onto the endoscope. An injection needle is passed through the working channel of the endoscope. When injection is performed appropriately into the submucosal layer, lifting of the mucosa (including the target lesion) can be achieved. The distal part of the lesion is lifted first. This ensures that the lesion is always kept in endoscopic view. (*C*) Prelooping of the snare wire. Snare wire is fixed to the rim of the distal attachment cap. (*D*) After creating the preloop, target mucosa is captured inside the cap. Full endoscopic suction draws the lifted mucosa inside the cap. Large-volume injection of saline avoids muscle involvement. (*E*) The lesion was caught by endoscopic suction inside distal attachment cap. (*F*) Snare wire is closed tightly. The captured mucosa looks like a pseudopolyp, which is resected by electrocautery. Coagulation current is the best option for achieving complete hemostasis. (*G*) Pseudopolyp that includes cancerous lesion was resected by electrocautery. This process is similar to conventional polypectomy. (*H*) Artificial ulcer was induced. Submucosal layer was observed as blue layer. (*I*) Resected specimen. A 9×5-mm lesion was resected in a single piece with enough lateral margin of nonneoplastic mucosa. (*J*) Esophageal squamous cell carcinoma. Cancer invaded deep submucosal layer (T1b). Invasion depth from lamina muscularis mucosa was 397 μm. In this case, cancer infiltration depth was SM2, which has a potential risk of approximately 40% lymph node involvement. This patient refused to receive surgery. Chemotherapy was carried out several times.

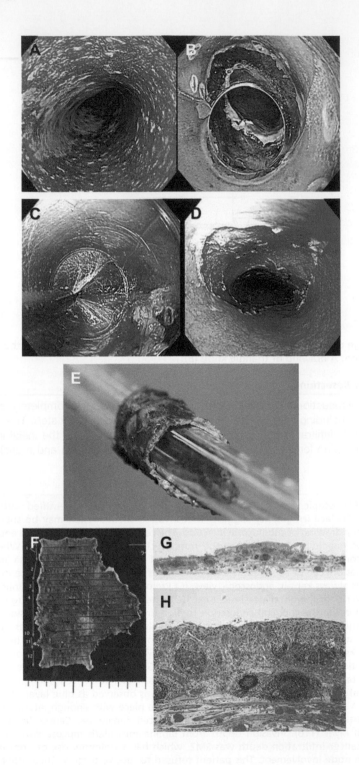

Repeated saline injection is therefore necessary to reduce the risk of muscle involvement during the procedure.[11]

ESD USING TT KNIFE

EMR is a technique originally based on a snare polypectomy. The procedure is simple and quick, but the size of the specimen resected by EMR is limited to around a maximum of 2 to 3 cm. ESD is a novel technique of endoscopic tissue resection that enables one-piece resection, regardless of size, even for a superficial widely spreading tumor. In ESD, a knife activated with electrocautery is used for the marginal cut and the submucosal dissection beneath the isolated mucosa. ESD was first developed by Ono and colleagues.[12] Subsequently, many additional devices have been designed and developed, and they are commercially available for ESD, including an insulation-tip knife, a hook knife, a flex knife, and a TT knife.[10,12–15]

TT Knife Procedure

ESD allows removal of the lesion in a single resection, even if the lesion is an extended one. The TT knife works as a multipurpose device for ESD (**Fig. 3**). ESD is a technique to resect mucosa using an electrocautery knife by dissecting submucosal connective tissue (**Fig. 4**). A key to perform safe ESD is to keep the muscle layer intact during the procedure. The tip of the TT knife is used to mark alongside the lesion margin. At this stage, the triangle plate is kept inside the outer sheath. Touching the tip of the outer sheath onto the mucosal surface is enough to mark with electrocautery current.

Marginal cut

The first step of dissection is marginal cutting alongside the lesion. Epinephrine/saline is injected to lift up the mucosa. A marginal cut is always achieved from the proximal margin to the distal end, and then circumferential cutting of the surrounding mucosa is completed (see **Fig. 4**B). Marginal cutting is done around 5 mm outside the marking. The TT knife hooks the mucosal edge and pulls up the target mucosa in the direction opposite from the surface of the muscle layer and then cuts it by electrocautery. By repeating the process, circumferential cutting of the target mucosa is completed.

◄───────

Fig. 4. (A) Chromoendoscopy with Lugol solution. Cancerous lesion was clearly demonstrated as an uncolored area. (B) Endoscopic image during ESD. Circumferential cut of the distal margin was done using TT knife. (C) Endoscopic image during ESD. Submucosal dissection using triangle-tip knife. Submucosal connective tissue was captured and then cut. Muscle layer surface is observed at the top of the image. Dissected specimen is observed at the bottom of the image. (D) Endoscopic image just after ESD. Proximal end of circumferentially induced artificial ulcer is observed. (E) Resected specimen was fixed on a transparent tube. Single-piece resection was completed even for almost circumferential lesion. (F) Photograph of the resected specimen. Resected specimen was divided into 2-mm columns. Mapping on the specimen was done. Red lines demonstrate M1 infiltration of cancer. Black lines demonstrate M2 infiltration of cancer. M1: cancer invasion is confined with epithelial layer. M2: cancer invades into proper mucosal layer but invasion does not reach lamina muscularis mucosae. (G) Histopathological image. Lower power magnification. In the area of M2 infiltration epithelial surface was elevated. (H) Histopathological image. Moderate power magnification. In the area of M2 infiltration cancer tissue is invaded into proper mucosal layer, but does not invade to lamina musclaris mucosal. M1 and M2 cancer has approximately no risk of lymph node metastasis, and then ESD is considered to be a curative treatment.

Submucosal dissection

The second step is submucosal dissection. Injection with a high-viscosity solution is mandatory to accomplish this process because it maintains mucosal lifting for a longer time. The authors now use hyaluronic acid for injection. The energy source is also an important factor in performing ESD safely. Swift coagulation 50W effect 3 (Vio 300D, ERBE USA Inc, Marietta, GA, USA) is now considered to be the best match for the TT knife. Submucosal dissection using the tip of the TT knife is subsequently carried out (see **Fig. 4**C). The hood mounted on the tip of the endoscope creates a working space beneath the mucosa and provides countertraction to the tissue in the submucosa. After removal of the mobilized mucosa, complete hemostasis is achieved by using the coagulation forceps (see **Fig. 4**D).

WHICH PROCEDURE SHOULD BE APPLIED?

Generally, a small lesion can be easily excised by the EMR-C procedure. In the esophagus, lesions less than 2 cm are resected by 1 session of EMR-C. ESD with TT knife is applied to larger lesions for en bloc resection.

CLINICAL RESULTS AND COMPLICATIONS OF EMR/ESD

Potential complications of EMR and ESD procedures include bleeding, perforation, and stricture. Bleeding can generally be managed with standard hemostatic techniques, including the use of endoclips. Perforation is rare and may be treated by surgery, endoscopic clipping, or conservative treatment.

The EMR-C procedure has been applied to 412 cases (222 in the esophagus and 190 in the stomach) in the upper gastrointestinal tract. ESD with the TT knife was developed in 2002 and has already been applied to 78 cases (13 in the esophagus and 63 in the stomach). Perforation occurred in 1 case in the esophagus and in 7 cases in the stomach. Perforation in the esophagus occurred on the fifth postoperative day and was successfully treated by conservative therapy. Procedure-related mortality was nil in a total of 490 cases in which EMR or ESD was applied.

COMPLETE REMOVAL OF BARRETT MUCOSA WITH HIGH-GRADE DYSPLASIA IN THE DISTAL ESOPHAGUS AND CARDIA

In Japan, the incidence of Barrett esophagus and Barrett esophageal carcinoma are relatively lower than in Western countries. The authors have performed a total of 8 EMR-C procedures for superficial carcinoma arising in Barrett esophagus. All cases were successfully treated solely with EMR, without any major complications. One-piece resection with ESD for focal adenocarcinoma arising on long-segment Barrett esophagus was carried out in 3 cases, and local control was excellent. This is the authors' first case of performing circumferential EMR for long-segment Barrett esophagus, and this is the first report describing total circumferential EMR for Barrett esophageal carcinoma. Total removal of long-segment Barrett with piecemeal EMR technique was already reported.[16]

May and colleagues[17] described a large series of patients managed with local endoscopic therapy for intraepithelial high-grade dysplasia and early adenocarcinoma in Barrett esophagus. The overall complication rate was 9.5%, and the calculated 3-year survival was 88%. On the basis of the result, local endoscopic therapy seems to be an effective and safe alternative to esophagectomy for the treatment of high-grade dysplasia and early-stage adenocarcinoma.

Ablative therapy, for instance, with photodynamic therapy,[18] has also been used as an alternative to surgical therapy, but there may be several limitations to ablative therapy compared with EMR/ESD. Adenocarcinoma may persist beneath reepithelialized squamous epithelial tissue.[19] In addition, EMR/ESD permits staging of the neoplastic change, because they allow detection of occult carcinoma or areas of invasion that are not suspected on the basis of endoscopic biopsy and endoscopic ultrasonography.

It has been proposed that EMR/ESD should be limited to within three-quarters of the circumference of the esophagus and that near-total or total mucosal resection should be avoided owing to refractory stenosis after healing of the resulting ulcer.[20]

Possible approaches may include 2-stage full-circumference resection at an interval of 8 weeks[1,20] or ablative therapy. When circumferential mucosal resection is performed with this technique on long-segment Barrett esophagus, multiple specimens are obtained, making precise reconstruction of the resected specimens extremely difficult. This may be theoretically averted by ESD to acquire one-piece specimen for better histologic analysis.

SUMMARY

EMR and ESD allow total removal of local lesions and precise histopathologic evaluation of the resected specimen, which helps to decide on additional treatment intending complete cure of the disease.

REFERENCES

1. Makuuchi H. Endoscopic mucosal resection for early esophageal cancer. Dig Endosc 1996;8:175–9.
2. Monma K, Sakaki N, Yoshida M. Endoscopic mucosectomy for precise evaluation and treatment of esophageal intraepithelial cancer. Dig Endosc 1990;2:447–52.
3. Inoue H, Endo M. Endoscopic esophageal mucosal resection using a transparent tube. Surg Endosc 1990;4:198–201.
4. Inoue H. Endoscopic mucosal resection for gastrointestinal mucosal cancers. In: Classen M, Tytgat GNJ, Lightdale C, editors. Gastroenterological endoscopy. Stuttgart, New York: Thieme; 2000. p. 322–33.
5. Endo M, Takeshita K, Yoshida M. How can we diagnose the early stage of esophageal cancer? Endoscopy 1986;18:11–8.
6. Lambert R. Diagnosis of esophagogastric tumors. Endoscopy 2004;36:110–9.
7. Seewald S, Ang TL, Soehendra N. Endoscopic mucosal resection of Barrett's esophagus containing dysplasia or intramucosal cancer. Postgrad Med J 2007; 83:367–72.
8. Vieth M, Ell C, Gossner L, et al. Histological analysis of endoscopic resection specimens for 326 patients with Barrett's esophagus and early neoplasia. Endoscopy 2004;36:776–81.
9. Inoue H, Takeshita K, Hori H, et al. Endoscopic mucosal resection with a cap-fitted panendoscpe for esophagus, stomach, and colon mucosal lesions. Gastrointest Endosc 1993;39:58–62.
10. Inoue H, Satoh Y, Sugaya S, et al. Endoscopic mucosal resection for early-stage gastrointestinal cancers. Best Pract Res Clin Gastroenterol 2005;19:871–87.
11. Inoue H, Kawano T, Tani M, et al. Endoscopic mucosal resection using a cap: technique for use and preventing perforation. Can J Gastroenterol 1999;13: 477–80.

12. Ono H, Kondo H, Gotoda T, et al. Endoscopic mucosal resection for treatment of early gastric cancer. Gut 2001;48:225–9.
13. Yamamoto H, Yube T, Isoda N, et al. A novel method of endoscopic mucosal resection using sodium hyaluronate. Gastrointest Endosc 1999;50:251–6.
14. Oyama T, Kikuchi Y. Aggressive endoscopic mucosal resection in the upper GI tract—hook knife EMR method. Minim Invasive Ther Allied Technol 2002;11: 291–5.
15. Yahagi N, Fujishiro M, Iguchi M, et al. Theoretical and technical requirements to expand EMR indications. Dig Endosc 2003;15:S19–21.
16. Satodate H, Inoue H, Yoshida T, et al. Circumferential EMR of carcinoma arising in Barrett's esophagus: case report. Gastrointest Endosc 2003;58:288–92.
17. May A, Gossner L, Pech O, et al. Local endoscopic therapy for intraepithelial high-grade neoplasia and early adenocarcinoma in Barrett's esophagus: acute-phase and long-term results of new treatment approach. Eur J Gastroenterol Hepatol 2002;14:1085–91.
18. Overholt BF, Panjehpour M, Haydek JM. Photodynamic therapy for Barrett's esophagus: follow-up in 100 patients. Gastrointest Endosc 1999;49:1–7.
19. Sampliner RE, Fass R. Partial regression of Barrett's esophagus: an inadequate endpoint. Am J Gastroenterol 1993;88:2092–4.
20. Inoue H, Kudo S. Endoscopic mucosal resection for gastrointestinal mucosal cancer. In: Meinhard C, Guido NJ, Charles JL, editors. Gastroenterological endoscopy. New York: Thieme; 2002. p. 322–33.

The Role of Photodynamic Therapy in the Esophagus

Seth A. Gross, MD[a], Herbert C. Wolfsen, MD[b,c],*

KEYWORDS

- Porfimer sodium • Aminolevulinic acid • HPPH (Photochlor)
- mTHPC (Foscan) • Subsquamous Barrett glands

Although the photodynamic effect has been known since ancient times, the modern use of photodynamic therapy (PDT) was not discovered until the early 20th century. Dougherty and colleagues[1] were the first to describe the response of malignancies to PDT, using hematoporphyrin derivative (HpD) exposure to red light.

The US Food and Drug Administration (FDA) did not approve the use of porfimer sodium PDT (Ps-PDT) for the palliation of patients with obstructing esophagus cancer until 1995. In 2003, Ps-PDT was granted regulatory approval as an alternative to esophagectomy for patients with Barrett esophagus and high-grade dysplasia (BE-HGD).

PDT is a complex treatment, and several components are necessary to achieve a tumor-destructive effect. The photosensitizer accumulates in malignant and premalignant tissue before light activation therapy. The most common photosensitizer is porfimer sodium, which is injected at a dose of 1.5 to 2 mg/kg 24 to 72 hours before the procedure. Other commonly used photosensitizers include m-tetrahydroxyphenyl chlorine (mTHPC) and aminolevulinic acid (ALA). Porfimer sodium is aromatically complex and becomes active when exposed to light at a wavelength of 630 nm. The excited molecules then react with oxygen, resulting in singlet oxygen and other reactive oxygen species, which leads to cell-membrane damage and ultimately apoptosis. The depth of invasion at wavelength of 630 nm is estimated to be 5 to 6 mm, depending on tissue blood flow and oxygen levels. The patient returns for upper endoscopy, using a diffusing light fiber placed alongside the targeted tissue, within an estimated 48 hours of injecting the photosensitizer. Patients may subsequently return

Funding support: none.

Financial disclosure: no financial disclosures or conflicts of interest to report.

a Division of Gastroenterology, Norwalk Hospital, Maple Street, Norwalk, CT 06856, USA

b Division of Gastroenterology and Hepatology, Mayo Clinic Florida, 4500 San Pablo Road, Jacksonville, FL 32224, USA

c Department of Medicine, Mayo Clinic College of Medicine, Rochester, MN, USA

* Corresponding author.

E-mail address: wolfsen.herbert@mayo.edu (H.C. Wolfsen).

Gastrointest Endoscopy Clin N Am 20 (2010) 35–53

doi:10.1016/j.giec.2009.07.008

1052-5157/09/$ – see front matter © 2010 Elsevier Inc. All rights reserved.

giendo.theclinics.com

within 24 to 48 hours for repeated laser light application to make sure the targeted area is completely treated.[2]

This review of PDT focuses on its role in the treatment of esophageal dysplasia and carcinoma, including some of the best tested and earliest clinical applications to receive regulatory approval. Initially, most of this research focused on the use of Ps-PDT in patients with advanced esophageal cancer,[3–5] leading to regulatory approvals in Japan, North America, United Kingdom, and mainland Europe. Later, multicenter studies examined the use of Ps-PDT in BE-HGD patients,[6,7] including a prospective, randomized, controlled international trial that demonstrated a significantly reduced rate of development of invasive carcinoma. These studies, and many others, established the importance of Ps-PDT in the treatment of esophageal dysplasia and neoplasia and supported the development and clinical use of other photosensitizers (**Table 1**).[8–15]

Key differences among these studies were patient selection, diagnostic evaluation, and PDT methods (ie, the photosensitizer, and its dose and route of administration). The light wavelength is particularly important since red light at 630 nm penetrates the esophageal tissue more deeply than green light at 532 nm. It is critical to note the other methods of ablation used in the study, and the rigor of postablation endoscopic surveillance. Although regulatory trials allow the use of PDT only, clinical series frequently use "focal" ablation methods (such as radiofrequency energy, argon plasma coagulation, or low-pressure liquid nitrogen cryotherapy) to remove small amounts of residual BE that persist after the initial PDT procedure. Regardless of treatment modality, it is recommended that all Barrett glandular metaplasia and dysplasia be removed to prevent the development or recurrence of invasive carcinoma.

BE-HGD AND EARLY CANCER

The incidence of esophageal carcinoma, particularly in Western developed countries, has steadily increased in the past 50 years.[16–22] BE is known to be the most important risk factor in the development of dysplasia and progression to esophageal adenocarcinoma.[6,23–29] Endoscopic ablation therapy such as PDT is an ideal treatment for esophageal diseases, including BE, as gastrointestinal endoscopy provides ready access to the target mucosa for laser light application. Depending on the photosensitizer selected, the wavelength, and the dose of light energy used, PDT permits deep mucosal penetration of light energy to drive the photodynamic reaction with little risk of perforation, despite the relatively thin esophageal mucosa and its limited blood supply.[30]

After the initial description of porphyrin-based PDT, HpD and dihematoporphyrin ether (DHE) activated with red light were the most commonly used photosensitizers.[31] Subsequently, these drugs were better purified and characterized for commercial production in the form of porfimer sodium (Photofrin, Axcan Scandipharm, Mont-Saint-Hilaire, Quebec, Canada).[32] Surgeons and gastrointestinal endoscopists used the prolonged mucosal retention of porfimer sodium, combined with red light activation, for deep mucosal and submucosal necrosis in the palliative treatment of advanced, obstructing lesions, and for the complete destruction of early cancers. The initial clinical studies were performed in patients with advanced carcinoma, and the results were compared with endoscopic palliation using stents or tumor ablation with thermal lasers. Improved endoscopic light delivery and dosimetry led to the use of Ps-PDT in patients with esophageal dysplasia (squamous dysplasia and BE with dysplasia).

Table 1
Types of photosensitizers for esophageal PDT

Class	Photosensitizer	Treatment Wavelength (λ, nm)	Diagnostic Fluorescence Wavelength (λ, nm)	Comments
Porphyrins	Porfimer sodium; also HpD; DHE	630	665–690	Porfimer sodium excellent red light tissue penetration with risk of stricture and prolonged skin sensitivity (Photofrin; also Photosan)
	5-ALA, a precursor of endogenous porphyrins	630–635	525, 665–690	Limited tissue penetration (≤2 mm); less photosensitivity (Levulan; Metvix)
Chlorins	mTHPC; temoporfin	650–660 (red) 514 (green)	525	Highly selective, potent 514 (green) compound suitable for less powerful light sources. Approved in European Union, Norway and Iceland (Foscan; Biolitec Pharma)
Purpurins (porphyrin macromolecules)	Mono-L-aspartyl chlorine e6 (NPe6; talaporfin or LS11); tin-etio-purpurin (SnEt2)	660–665	675	Phase III study using LS11 for hepatoma activated with light emitting diode (LED) (Light Sciences Oncology, Bellevue, WA, USA[93])
Phthalocyanine	Silicon phthalocyanine (Pc4); aluminum disulfonated phthalocyanine (AlSPc); chloroaluminum phthalocyanine tetrasulfonate (AlPcS4)	675	610	Limited phototoxicity and limited clinical information hydrophobic compounds that are difficult to purify. Selective tumor retention, minimal dark and cutaneous photosensitivity and excellent photodynamic activity are expected (Photosens)
Benzoporphyrins	Benzoporphyrin derivative (BPD); benzoporphyrin derivative monoacid (BPDMA); diethylene glycol benzoporphyrin derivative (Lemuteporfin)	690	690	Rapid tumor accumulation; transient limited skin photosensitivity and prominent vascular effects produced approval for use in macular degeneration (Visudyne); new diethylene glycol functionalized chlorine-type photosensitizer[94]
Porphyrin-like compounds	Motexafin lutetium; lutetium texaphyrin	730–740	730–740	Rapid tissue uptake and clearance and tissue penetration; used for photochemical angioplasty (Antrin, Lutrin, Lu-Tex)
Pheophorbides (tetrapyriolea) chlorophyll derivatives	2-[1-Hexyloxyethyl]-2-devinyl-pyropheophorbide-a (HPPH)	680	680	Undergoing evaluations for use in esophageal, skin, and recurrent breast cancer (Photochlor)

Despite these advantages, porfimer sodium remains a first-generation drug that is relatively inefficient and produces prolonged photosensitivity, typically lasting 4 to 6 weeks. More recently developed photosensitizer agents include mTHPC (temoporfin, Foscan, Biolitec AG, Jena, Germany), a potent photosensitizing agent that requires lower drug and light doses and induces only 2 to 3 weeks of cutaneous photosensitivity. However, studies using mTHPC have been associated with higher stricture formation or full-thickness tissue necrosis and perforation. Another photosensitizing agent, ALA, is converted within the gut mucosa to its active form protoporphyrin IX (PpIX), and accumulates in the mucosal layer of the gut,[33] which decreases the risk of stricture formation by sparing damage to the deeper esophageal wall and muscle layers.[34] Commercially available preparations of ALA include aminolevulinic acid (Levulan, DUSA Pharmaceuticals, Wilmington, MA, USA), δ-aminolevulinic acid (medac GmbH, Wedel, Germany) and methyl aminolevulinate (Metvix, Photocure ASA, Oslo, Norway). Clinical experience with ALA in the esophagus has produced varied results, particularly in controlled trials performed with other forms of thermal ablation. 2-[1-Hexyloxyethyl]-2-devinyl-pyro-pheophorbide-a (HPPH, or Photochlor), a pheophorbide photosensitizer owned by the Roswell Park Cancer Institute. It features only mild photosensitivity at antitumor doses, but has not yet been widely tested in clinical studies.[35] A more complete listing of photosensitizers used in esophageal PDT is given in **Table 1**.

PORFIMER SODIUM AND HPD

Porfimer sodium is the most widely used photosensitizer in clinical practice and gastroenterological PDT. Porfimer sodium, an HpD, first received regulatory approval in Canada (1994), and then in the United States and Europe (1995), for the treatment of patients with advanced esophageal carcinoma.[36] Overholt and colleagues[37] reported the use of Ps-PDT in 84 BE patients who had low-grade dysplasia (LGD) or HGD and in 14 patients with T1 adenocarcinoma, with a mean follow-up of 19 months. To obtain improved light dosimetry and more uniform light-energy application, a balloon fiber centering device with mirrored caps was used to distend and flatten the esophageal mucosa. These investigators found that BE and LGD were eliminated in 92% of patients, and HGD was eliminated in 88% of patients. Complete elimination of Barrett glandular mucosa was noted in 43% of patients. In the group of patients with early cancer, successful endoscopic ablation was confirmed in 10 out of 14 cancers. The most common post-PDT complication was stricture development (34% of patients). It was often more common in those patients who had more than one session of PDT. Over the 19 months mean follow-up of this study, subsquamous epithelium was detected in 6% of patients, but there were no signs of dysplasia or cancer.

Several other centers with large clinical series subsequently reported similar results, with emphasis on the diagnostic evaluation of patients with esophageal dysplasia, including the use of endoscopic mucosal resection and endoscopic ultrasound with fine-needle aspiration for lymphadenopathy.[13,38,39] Wolfsen and colleagues[40] reviewed their experience treating 102 BE-HGD patients (n = 69) or early cancer patients (n = 33) with PDT, during a mean follow-up of 1.6 years. Fifty-six percent of patients had complete ablation of Barrett glandular epithelium, with a single session of Ps-PDT. Treatment failure was detected in four patients, with persistent HGD or carcinoma that required subsequent curative esophagectomy. A combined Mayo Clinic study at two independent sites enrolled 142 patients (60 patients at Jacksonville, Florida, and 72 patients at Rochester, Minnesota) for treatment with Ps-PDT, and followed these patients for a mean of 19 months.[41,42] Complete elimination of BE was noted in 50% and 35% of patients, respectively. A balloon centering device was not used during the treatment sessions. Any residual disease detected after Ps-PDT was treated with argon plasma coagulation (APC), resulting in elimination of HGD in 100% and 80% of patients, respectively. The rates of post-PDT complications and stricture formation were 20% and 27%, respectively, rates comparable to those previously reported by Overholt.[37] There was also a transient weight loss in patients who suffered from post-PDT chest discomfort or odynophagia.[43] The number of patients who reported experiencing cutaneous photosensitivity was similar in the Minnesota and Florida patients.[44] The rate of residual subsquamous epithelium was 0% and 4%, respectively, and 4% (n = 5) had residual dysplasia or neoplasm, ultimately requiring curative esophagectomy. In an effort to reduce the rate of stricture formation, a group of 60 patients with BE-HGD were treated with PDT alone or PDT combined with oral prednisone, but this strategy did not impact the rate of stricture formation. In the group given PDT alone, the stricture rate was 16% compared with 29% when PDT was combined with prednisone.[45] Updated studies have compared the results of Ps-PDT alone and combined with endoscopic mucosal resection, and in a comparative cohort study with patients who have undergone esophagectomy. These studies found a similar overall survival in patients treated with endoscopic therapy using electromagnetic radiation and PS-PDT compared with surgery.[46,47] The General Infirmary at Leeds, UK and the University of Pittsburgh Medical Center, Pittsburgh, Pennsylvania, reported similar efficacy in patients with BE-HGD and esophageal carcinoma. Foroulis and Thorpe[48] retrospectively evaluated the effectiveness of Ps-PDT in 31 patients with BE-HGD, 10 patients with intramucosal carcinoma, and 6 patients with endosonography stage T2 carcinoma, during a median follow-up of 10 months. In patients with HGD or intramucosal cancer, the treatment response was 80.9%. In patients with more advanced disease (T1b/T2), 2 of the 6 patients who were unfit for surgical resection had a complete response. Keeley and colleagues[49] reviewed their experience using Ps-PDT in 50 patients treated for BE-HGD (13 patients) or locally advanced carcinoma, with a mean follow-up of 28 months. Sixteen patients also received treatment with chemoradiation. At last follow-up, 16 patients were alive and disease free, and 15 patients were receiving additional treatment for persistent or recurrent disease. The study concluded that Ps-PDT was potentially curative for patients with BE-HGD and superficial esophageal carcinomas, but not for more advanced disease.

The Photodynamic Therapy for Barrett's Esophagus (PHO-BAR) trial was the first multicenter randomized control trial to evaluate the utility of Ps-PDT in patients with BE-HGD to be approved by the FDA. The study involved 30 sites, used an expert centralized pathology laboratory, and studied 208 patients randomized to PDT plus omeprazole or omeprazole alone (20 mg twice daily). After the initial treatment with Ps-PDT at 12 months, 41% of patients had complete remission of BE, and 72% had complete elimination of BE-HGD. This was statistically significant compared with the group with omeprazole alone. Treatment with Ps-PDT also decreased the rate of progression to adenocarcinoma from 28% in the drug-only group, to less than 10% in the PDT-plus-omeprazole group. These results were maintained at 2 years follow-up, resulting in the approval of Ps-PDT for treatment of BE-HGD in North America, United Kingdom, mainland Europe, and Japan. Recently, Overholt and colleagues[7] reported a 5-year follow-up of the original study. They found persistent successful elimination of BE-HGD significantly more often in patients from the Ps-PDT-plus-omeprazole group (77%), compared with 39% of patients in the omeprazole-alone group. The secondary outcome of progressing to cancer remained significantly lower (15%) in the Ps-PDT-plus-omeprazole group compared with 29% in the omeprazole-alone group. Based on these large single-center studies with long-term follow-up and the results of this randomized controlled trial, porfimer sodium has become a first-line therapy for treating BE-HGD and superficial carcinoma at many referral centers.[50–52] Although Ps-PDT has been shown to be efficacious in the treatment of BE-HGD, neo-squamous overgrowth of Barrett mucosa may mask persistent dysplasia or cancer (so-called buried Barrett). Bronner and colleagues[53] analyzed the histologic specimens of 33,658 biopsies from the PHO-BAR study and found no differences in squamous over-growth between the 2 patient groups (those treated with acid-blocker therapy only and those treated with Ps-PDT). Long term studies found no risk of missing subsquamous dysplasia or carcinoma.

Stricture formation is the most common side effect with Ps-PDT. The pathophys-iology of stricture development is not known. It has been postulated that the deep burn of Ps-PDT causes an inflammatory reaction, leading to a fibrotic response, re-sulting in stricture formation. Yachimski and colleagues[54] retrospectively tried to identify pretreatment variables that may lead to postablation stricture development. One-hundred and sixteen patients had a total of 160 sessions of PDT, but only 16% of patients experienced stricture after their initial treatment. Patients having a second PDT treatment had overall stricture rate of 23%. Stricture development was not related to age, gender, body mass index, or prior endoscopic mucosal resection. Independent predictors of stricture development included patients with a longer segment, multiple PDT treatments, and evidence of intramucosal carci-noma before PDT. However, there is wide variation in Ps-PDT treatment parame-ters; a recent study compared pretreatment evaluation protocols, PDT light dosimetry, and follow-up evaluation protocols, in 10 large PDT referral centers in the United States.[8]

mTHPC

The chlorine derivative mTHPC is an efficient photosensitizer that has been used in Europe, mostly for the treatment of advanced head and neck cancer.[55] A large US trial performed in patients with head and neck squamous cell carcinoma was complicated by treatment-associated tissue necrosis, tissue breakdown, and stricture formation. This highly selective photosensitizer is associated with photosensitivity that lasts for only 2 to 3 weeks after administration. In a limited number of gastroenterologic studies, mTHPC has been administered intravenously at a dosage of 0.15 mg/kg with 652 nm light activation.[56] Gossner and colleagues[57–59] have used mTHPC as salvage therapy in a small number of BE-HGD patients in whom previous treatment with ALA-PDT failed. Javaid and colleagues[60] treated 4 patients with BE-HGD using mTHPC and an argon-pump dye laser light of 652 nm and 2 patients using a xenon arc lamp (Paterson-Whitehurst lamp, 652 nm), with equivalent results, demonstrating that efficient photosensitizers do not require high-power laser light sources for effec-tive activation. Etienne and colleagues[61] used mTHPC with green light PDT in 12 BE-HGD patients and 7 patients with mucosal esophageal carcinoma. There was a mean follow-up of 34 months, with only an 8% recurrence of disease. Lovat and colleagues[62] conducted a pilot study to assess the efficacy of mTHPC, including 7 patients with BE-HGD and 12 patients with superficial esophageal cancer. Treatment results were variable, but much better for patients treated with red light, including successful ablation in 4 of 6 carcinoma patients and 3 of 4 BE-HGD patients. None of the patients treated with green light experienced successful disease eradication or reached long-term remission.

This limited experience demonstrates that although mTHPC is a potent photosen-sitizer, it is able to eliminate columnar epithelium in the esophagus and downgrade the degree of dysplasia, but the optimal light and drug dosimetry are unknown. Further studies are required to determine ideal treatment parameters to avoid excessive tissue necrosis and high rates of stricture.

ALA

As described earlier in this article, ALA is a prodrug that stimulates the endogenous production of PpIX, mostly within the gut mucosa. ALA and Metvix brands have been used for several years, mostly in Europe, including Scandinavia. Levulan, a commercially available form of ALA, was recently granted orphan drug status by the FDA for the treatment of patients with BE-HGD. This unusual decision comes after recent approvals for treatment of BE using Ps-PDT, radiofrequency energy ablation, and low-pressure liquid nitrogen cryotherapy ablation. Regardless, ALA has previously been used for PDT in the United Kingdom and mainland Europe for BE with dysplasia and superficial carcinoma. ALA is considered a second-generation porphyrin-type photosensitizer. It is activated using red light (635 nm) and offers several advantages, including targeting the superficial mucosal layer and a shortened photosensitivity lasting only 24 to 48 hours.[63–66] The initial randomized double-blind placebo-controlled trial was conducted in the United Kingdom for patients with Barrett LGD. ALA-PDT was given orally at a dose of 30 mg/kg and activated by a green light (514 nm), to enhance superficial mucosal damage and limit the risk of stricture formation.[67,68] Patients were followed for a mean of 24 months, and there was an endoscopic response in 83% of patients. After ablation, surveillance endoscopy with biopsies demonstrated that 98% of the patients were dysplasia free, with only a single case of recurrent LGD, in a 12-month follow-up. These encouraging results were also seen by other researchers treating BE-HGD.[57,59,69,70] A group in Wiesbaden, Germany, has published several studies using ALA-PDT in patients with BE-HGD and superficial carcinoma; it is presumed that the authors describe studies from the same cohort of patients. Pech reported the treatment of 35 BE-HGD patients using ALA-PDT. They noted a high complete response rate in 97% of patients, at a mean follow-up of 42 months.[71] A follow-up study examined 66 patients with BE-HGD (n = 35) or an early adenocarcinoma (n = 31). ALA was administered orally at a dose of 60 mg/kg 4 to 6 hours before endoscopy with laser light application, using light between 630 and 635 nm with an energy dose of 150 J/cm. Follow-up endoscopy procedures used argon beam coagulation or thermal potassium titanyl phosphate laser to destroy any residual glandular mucosa. An intensive endoscopic surveillance program scheduled endoscopy at 1, 2, 3, 6, 9, and 12 months, with procedures every 6 months thereafter for 5 years. During a follow-up period, with a mean of 37 months, 97% of patients with BE-HGD and 100% of early cancer patients achieved a complete response. Disease recurrence was detected in one patient with BE-HGD (89% disease-free survival), and in 10 carcinoma patients (68% disease-free survival). However, no deaths related to Barrett neoplasia were reported.[71,72] From the same group, Behrens and May recently reported complete remission with the combined use of endoscopic mucosal resection, ALA-PDT, and argon beam coagulation in 44 and 49 patients, respectively.[73,74] PDT using orally administered ALA has been associated with adverse effects such as significant chest pain, elevated liver enzyme tests, acute neuropathy mimicking porphyria, and sudden death, presumably related to cardiac dysrhythmia.[75] Although considered by some to be only of minor importance, most ALA-PDT treatment occurs in the hospital setting for safety reasons and pain control.[76]

Ortner and colleagues[77] attempted to avoid the risks of systemic ALA administration by using the drug topically, with 15 or 60 mg/kg body weight in an 8.5% sodium bicarbonate solution in saline, using a spray catheter during endoscopy, in 7 patients with

Barrett metaplasia and 7 patients with Barrett LGD. Although it was safe and effective in ablating LGD in all 7 patients, a patient with metaplasia progressed to HGD after treatment. Complete ablation of all BE was noted in only 21% of patients after the initial PDT, and in 20% after the second PDT. Therefore, topical administration of ALA was not a reliable method of ablation in these patients. Several small randomized trials have been performed using ALA-PDT in patients with Barrett metaplasia or LGD. ALA-PDT has performed poorly in studies that compared its use with another endoscopic ablation treatment. Specifically, Ragunath and colleagues[78] studied 26 patients with Barrett dysplasia (23 with LGD, 3 with HGD) and found that the use of argon beam coagulation was more effective, less expensive, and associated with fewer complications, compared with ALA-PDT. Similar disappointing results were reported in a study in Sheffield of 68 patients with Barrett metaplasia and in a study from Adelaide, South Australia, in which 30 patients with Barrett LGD were treated with 30 mg/kg of ALA. In the Australian study, the ALA outcomes compared well with those of patients treated with APC.[67,79,80] A trial in Rotterdam was the only positive randomized trial. The investigators used 60 mg/kg ALA for PDT in 40 Barrett patients (32 metaplasia, 8 LGD), and compared ALA to APC. While successful reversal of BE was achieved in more than 3 patients in the study, multiple courses of therapy were required, and one ALA-PDT patient died of sudden death. The authors did not recommend those treatments for "prophylactic ablation of BE."[80,81] In a study in Amsterdam published the same year, 20 patients who had BE-HGD that persisted after endoscopic mucosal resections were treated with ALA-PDT (40 mg/kg).[82] The authors defined complete remission as the absence of BE-HGD in biopsies, taken at 2 surveillance endoscopy procedures. After ALA-PDT, all patients had persistent BE (median regression was 50%), and 5 of 20 patients (25%) had persistent HGD at surveillance examinations after PDT. Subsequent follow-up procedures found recurrence of HGD or carcinoma in another four patients, from 6 to 15 months after PDT. These findings suggest that ALA-PDT may be unreliable for treating patients with advanced disease (HGD or carcinoma). Regardless of the initial therapy used, all BE must be destroyed at follow-up endoscopy procedures to prevent the development or recurrence of carcinoma. In May 2007, an abstract from Mackenzie and colleagues[83] presented the results of a dosimetry study of 72 patients with BE-HGD. They compared the use of red or green light with varying doses of ALA. The main treatment outcome was the development of cancer after ALA-PDT. In the patients treated using the higher doses of ALA (60 mg/kg) and higher energy red light (1000 J/cm), only 3% of patients were subsequently diagnosed with invasive carcinoma, at a follow-up of 36 months. However, in the other groups, a much higher rate of cancer development was noted (34%). These results were found in a subset of patients participating in a study of varying drug and light-energy doses, in which 14 patients (20%) progressed to cancer. In addition, there was no mention of concomitant acid-blocker therapy, which is important for the successful ablation of BE. If this is the optimal ALA, light dose, and wavelength, then perhaps it is time for a randomized controlled trial of Levulan PDT in combination with acid-blocker drugs, versus drug therapy alone, as was performed for Ps-PDT and is under way for radiofrequency ablation.[83]

PDT AND LIGHT DOSIMETRY AND DELIVERY SYSTEMS

The future of PDT depends on the development of improved photosensitizers and light dosimetry. However, the costs of drug discovery, clinical testing, and regulatory approval will likely impede the further development of photosensitizers in gastroenterology. Therefore, if PDT is to remain a viable endoscopic mucosal ablation treatment option, it is mandatory to improve light dosimetry.[84–87] Currently, there are no means available to determine the ideal dose of light required for PDT in an individual patient, and imperfect light dosimetry doses may lead to insufficient treatment, with residual dysplasia or carcinoma. Alternatively, excessive light dosing may result in severe mucosal damage and stricture formation. A recent pilot study compared porfimer sodium tissue uptake, light dose, and esophagus wall thickness with patient outcomes. Eleven patients were included in the study. Patients with a mean porfimer sodium content of 6.2 mg/kg and a mean total light dose of 278 J/cm had complete treatment. Patients with a mean porfimer sodium tissue content of 3.9 mg/kg, and a mean total light dose of 268 J/cm had an incomplete treatment. Patients who received complete treatment had lower esophageal wall thickness compared with the group with incomplete treatment. This is the first study to link esophageal wall thickness and treatment outcome.[88]

In order to better target dysplastic tissue, researchers have continued to develop photosensitizers and optical devices, such as lasers and arc lamps coupled to a light delivery system. The light delivery system is often a quartz light diffuser or a specialized modified diffuser placed under fluoroscopy that has been modified for endoscopic usage. Because of the natural peristalsis of the esophagus and respiratory motion of the chest, it can be challenging to maintain central positioning of the fiber within the esophagus, to achieve uniform light distribution.[57] The natural mucosal folds of the esophagus, in conjunction with esophageal peristalsis and respiratory movement, create areas of mucosa shielded from light exposure, leading to incomplete mucosal ablation. This has led to the development of more advanced light systems to include an adaptable device to shape the esophagus using an elastic catheter balloon.[89] The balloon catheter allows the fiber to be centered to provide an equal distribution to the treatment area by eliminating the "shadow phenomenon," resulting from the hill-and-valley effect of mucosal folds. Panjehpour and colleagues[90] were able to flatten the esophageal mucosa using a nonelastic balloon stabilizing device. The wall of the esophagus should not be overdistended, as decreased blood flow can lead to decreased effectiveness of PDT.[89,91] Prasad and colleagues[92] determined that risk factors for developing strictures after PDT included a history of prior esophageal stricture, performance of endoscopic mucosal resection before PDT, and more than one PDT light application treatment. The use of a balloon centering device was not statistically significant in reducing the development of strictures. To eliminate esophageal folds, the Swiss group used a rigid, large-diameter light distributor greater than 18 mm that also controlled esophageal peristalsis and respiratory motion.[93] The tissue drug level can vary in each patient, making it difficult to predict actual tissue damage. The use of advanced optical techniques such as fluorescence spectroscopy or optical coherence tomography may help assess drug levels at the level of the mucosa and the progression of the photodynamic reaction to improve PDT outcomes.[94–96]

The Role of Biomarkers and PDT

The purpose of endoscopic therapy in BE is to interrupt the sequence of progression from dysplasia to carcinoma. Success of endoscopic therapy is often based on tissue histology that demonstrates eradication of dysplasia and metaplasia. However, recurrence of disease, and progression to carcinoma, can occur in the "success" cases, defined as the successful ablation of Barrett mucosa. Several genetic abnormalities, such as p16 and p53, are considered cell cycle checkpoint genes. Mutations of these genes are seen in patients with BE.[97,98]

Prasad and colleagues[99] assessed biomarkers in patients with BE-HGD or early carcinoma after PDT. Post-PDT biomarkers were obtained at 9 months from

Table 2
PDT for Barrett dysplasia and carcinoma

Author	Patients	Sensitizer	Route of Administration	Dosage (mg/kg)	Interval (h)	Wavelength (nm)	Light Dosage (J/cm)	Complete Eradication Neoplasia (%)	Buried Barrett (%)	Stenosis (%)	Follow-up (months)	Recurrence (%)
Overholt et al[36]	100 (8 HGD, 9 LGD, 3 Ca)	Sodium porfimer	IV	2	48	630	125–250	88 HGD, 92 LGD, Ca 77	5 (2 HGD, 1 Ca)	34	19	23
Wolfsen et al[40]	102 (69 HGD, 33 Ca)	Sodium porfimer	IV	2	48, 72	630	150–225	96	4 (HGD)	20	19	6
Foroulis and Thorpe[48]	25 (15 HGD, 10 Ca)	Sodium porfimer	IV	2	24	630	200–250	81	20	6	14	18
Keeley et al[49]	50 (19 HGD, Ca 31)	Sodium porfimer	IV	2	48	630	300–400	37 HGD	NA	42	28.1	31 HGD
Overholt et al[6]	138 HGD	Sodium porfimer	IV	2	40–50	630	130	77	NA	36	43	13
Overholt et al[7]	48 HGD	Sodium porfimer	IV	2	40–50	630	130 + 50	77	NA	2	60	5
Javid et al[60]	7 (6 HGD, 1 Ca)	mTHPC	IV	0.15	96	652	8–20	100	NA	29	NA	0
Etienne et al[61]	14 (7 HGD, 7 Ca)	mTHPC	IV	0.15	96	514	75	100	0	29	34	8
Lovat et al[62]	19 (7 HGD, 12 Ca)	mTHPC	IV	0.15	72	514 or 652	7–75	42	21	11	24	75
Ackroyd et al[67]	18 LGD	5-ALA	Oral	30	4	514	60	98	0	0	24	NA
Barr et al[69]	5 HGD	5-ALA	Oral	60	4	630	50–150	100	40	0	26–44	NA
Pech et al[71]	51 (30 HGD, 21 Ca)	5-ALA	Oral	60	4–6	635	150	100	NA	0	38	24

Gossner et al[59]	32 (10 HGD, 22 Ca)	5-ALA	Oral	60	4-6	635	150	84	7	0	9.9	7
Peters et al[82]	20 (18 HGD, 2 Ca)	5-ALA	Oral	40	1.5-4	630	100	75	53	0	30	27
Tan et al[106]	12 (2 HGD, 10 Ca)	5-ALA	Oral	60 or 75	4-6	630	100-200	16.6	NA	0	NA	NA
Ortner et al[77]	7 LGD	5-ALA	Topical	15	1.5-2	632	90 and 100	21	NA	0	33	7
Kelty et al[80]	25 NDBE	5-ALA	Oral	30 or 60	4-6	635	85	0	24	0	1	NA
Kelty et al[79]	34 NDBE	5-ALA	Oral	30	4-6	635	85	50	24	0	12	NA
Mackenzie et al[107]	24 HGD	5-ALA	Oral	60	3-5	635	500-1000 (× 2)	38	46	0	45 (1-78)	25 Ca
Ackroyd et al[108]	40 LGD	5-ALA	Oral	30	4	514	60	97	NA	0	53 (18-68)	3 Ca
Prasad et al[47]	103 HGD	Sodium porfimer	IV	2	48	630	200	86		27	36	6.2
	26 DHE	Sodium porfimer	IV	4	48	630	200	86		27	36	6.2
Conio et al[21]	83 T, CA	Sodium porfimer	IV	2	48	630	250	92	NA	11	36	7

Abbreviations: HGD, high-grade dysplasia; LGD, low-grade dysplasia; Ca, Barrett carcinoma; NDBE, nondysplastic Barrett esophagus; ALA, aminolevulinic acid; mTHPC, m-tetrahydroxyphenyl chlorine; IV, intravenous, NA, not available.

31 patients with a mean Barrett segment of 5 cm. Fluorescence in situ hybridization (FISH) showed that 24 patients had no HGD based on post-PDT histology, and 18 of these patients were FISH negative and had no recurrence. Six patients in this group remained FISH positive, 2 of whom had recurrent disease. Seven patients still had HGD/early carcinoma on histology despite PDT, and 5 of these patients remained FISH positive. This study demonstrated the relationship between histology and biomarkers. It suggests that if a patient has no dysplasia after PDT and there is a loss of biomarkers, then the patient will be less likely to have recurrent disease.

Hornick and colleagues[100] studied the biologic characteristics of nonburied and buried BE in patients treated with PDT. Patients with nonburied BE, who did not have dysplasia before PDT, had elevated crypt proliferation and DNA abnormalities. Patients treated with PDT who had residual nonburied BE without dysplasia continued to have elevated crypt proliferation, but minimal DNA abnormalities. Patients with buried BE after PDT had decreased crypt proliferation, but normal DNA profiles.

Another study focused on p53 expression in patients with HGD who were not treated, and compared those results with the neosquamous mucosa seen in patients' status after PDT. A total of 23 patients were split into 2 groups. Patients in group 1 (n = 12) had HGD treated with PDT. Patients in group 2 (n = 10) did not have PDT ablation. Biopsies from both groups were stained for p53 protein expression and then scored on an immunohistochemistry scoring system, with a range of 0 for negative and 2 to 8 for positive samples. Patients who did not have PDT for HGD had a median score of 7, compared with a score of 4 for the post-PDT group. Lower p53 expression was seen in the treated group, suggesting a decreased risk of progression to carcinoma.[101]

Endoscopic ablative therapy for BE with dysplasia is a first-line treatment option. There seems to be a role for biomarkers to complement histology to help assess a patient's potential response to ablative therapy.

SUMMARY

PDT has been a critically important tool for the advancement of endoscopic therapy for esophageal dysplasia and superficial carcinoma (**Table 2**). Based on the long-term outcomes of large Ps-PDT studies, endoscopic ablation therapy has been proven safe and reliable for the treatment of esophageal dysplasia to prevent the development of invasive carcinoma. However, treatment results using all forms of PDT could be significantly improved with better photosensitizers and more sophisticated light dosimetry.[102] The use of PDT has also been diminished by the development of other forms of ablation, such as radiofrequency energy, as described in the recent publication from Shaheen and colleagues[103] that demonstrated excellent rates of successful ablation in BE patients with LGD and HGD with no photosensitivity and a 5% rate of stricture. We believe that PS-PDT will remain an important therapeutic option for patients with Barrett HGD, early carcinoma, and other diseases such as bile duct carcinoma.[104] The use of PS-PDT for BE-HGD has been compared with surgery and surveillance endoscopy in several outcome studies[51,105] that found PS-PDT to be a cost-effective therapy. The long-term treatment results for PS-PDT after mucosal resection for patients with HGD were compared with a similar cohort of patients who were treated with esophageal resection surgery. The PDT-treated patients were older, had poorer performance status, and longer BE segments, yet overall mortality was similar in both groups (8.5% mortality at median 63 months in surgery group, versus 9% mortality at mean 57 months). Although recurrent HGD was found in the PDT group, all patients were re-treated with endoscopic methods. None of the patient deaths in either group was related to esophageal cancer.[47]

As the move away from the use of PDT is likely the result of its side-effect profile (mainly stricture development and cutaneous photosensitivity), its future depends on improving treatment parameters and dosimetry to improve outcomes and minimize complications ("optimized PDT").

Efforts to improve outcomes and avoid the complications associated with PDT have focused on measuring and creating dosimetry adjustments for variation in esophageal wall thickness, especially the mucosa and submucosal layers, mucosal oxygenation and blood flow, and the content of photosensitizers in the target esophageal wall layers.[88] Development of dosimetry systems to monitor the effects of any esophageal ablation (hot, cold, or photochemical) is important and necessary to avoid complications related to incomplete ablation with persistent disease from undertreatment or the development of stricture or perforation from overtreatment.

ACKNOWLEDGMENTS

The authors would like to acknowledge Katherine Purcell for her expert work in developing this issue and for reviewing all the articles.

REFERENCES

1. Dougherty TJ, Kaufman JE, Goldfarb A, et al. Photoradiation therapy for the treatment of malignant tumors. Cancer Res 1978;38(8):2628–35.
2. Macdonald J, Dougherty T. Basic principles of photodynamic therapy. J Porphyrins Phthalocyanines 2001;5(2):105–29.
3. McCaughan JS Jr, Ellison EC, Guy JT, et al. Photodynamic therapy for esophageal malignancy: a prospective twelve-year study. Ann Thorac Surg 1996;62(4):1005–9.
4. Litle VR, Luketich JD, Christie NA, et al. Photodynamic therapy as palliation for esophageal cancer: experience in 215 patients. Ann Thorac Surg 2003;76(5): 1687–92 [discussion: 92–3].
5. Lightdale CJ, Heier SK, Marcon NE, et al. Photodynamic therapy with porfimer sodium versus thermal ablation therapy with Nd:YAG laser for palliation of esophageal cancer: a multicenter randomized trial. Gastrointest Endosc 1995; 42(6):507–12.
6. Overholt BF, Lightdale CJ, Wang KK, et al. Photodynamic therapy with porfimer sodium for ablation of high-grade dysplasia in Barrett's esophagus: international, partially blinded, randomized phase III trial. Gastrointest Endosc 2005;62(4): 488–98.
7. Overholt BF, Wang KK, Burdick JS, et al. Five-year efficacy and safety of photodynamic therapy with Photofrin in Barrett's high-grade dysplasia. Gastrointest Endosc 2007;66:460–8.
8. Wolfsen HC. Endoluminal therapy for Barrett's esophagus [abstract]. Gastrointest Endosc Clin N Am 2007;17(1):59–82.
9. Wolfsen HC. Present status of photodynamic therapy for high-grade dysplasia in Barrett's esophagus. J Clin Gastroenterol 2005;39(3):189–202.
10. Wolfsen HC. Carpe luz-seize the light: endoprevention of esophageal adenocarcinoma when using photodynamic therapy with porfimer sodium. Gastrointest Endosc 2005;62(4):499–503.
11. Wolfsen HC. Endoprevention of esophageal cancer: endoscopic ablation of Barrett's metaplasia and dysplasia. Expert Rev Med Devices 2005;2(6):713–23.
12. Prosst RL, Wolfsen HC, Gahlen J. Photodynamic therapy for esophageal diseases: a clinical update. Endoscopy 2003;35(12):1059–68.

13. Wang KK. Current status of photodynamic therapy of Barrett's esophagus. Gastrointest Endosc 1999;49(3 Pt 2):S20–3.
14. Overholt BF, Panjehpour M, Halberg DL. Photodynamic therapy for Barrett's esophagus with dysplasia and/or early stage carcinoma: long-term results. Gastrointest Endosc 2003;58(2):183–8.
15. Sampliner RE. Prevention of adenocarcinoma by reversing Barrett's esophagus with mucosal ablation. World J Surg 2003;27(9):1026–9.
16. Falk GW. Barrett's esophagus. Gastroenterology 2002;122(6):1569–91.
17. Cameron AJ, Zinsmeister AR, Ballard DJ, et al. Prevalence of columnar-lined (Barrett's) esophagus. Comparison of population-based clinical and autopsy findings. Gastroenterology 1990;99(4):918–22.
18. Cameron AJ, Ott BJ, Payne WS. The incidence of adenocarcinoma in columnar-lined (Barrett's) esophagus. N Engl J Med 1985;313(14):857–9.
19. Reid BJ. Barrett's esophagus and esophageal adenocarcinoma. Gastroenterol Clin North Am 1991;20(4):817–34.
20. Ward EM, Wolfsen HC, Achem SR, et al. Barrett's esophagus is common in older men and women undergoing screening colonoscopy regardless of reflux symptoms. Am J Gastroenterol 2006;101(1):12–7.
21. Conio M, Lapertosa G, Blanchi S, et al. Barrett's esophagus: an update. Crit Rev Oncol Hematol 2003;46(2):187–206.
22. Devesa SS, Blot WJ, Fraumeni JF Jr. Changing patterns in the incidence of esophageal and gastric carcinoma in the United States. Cancer 1998;83(10):2049–53.
23. Montgomery E, Bronner MP, Goldblum JR, et al. Reproducibility of the diagnosis of dysplasia in Barrett esophagus: a reaffirmation. Hum Pathol 2001;32(4):368–78.
24. Buttar NS, Wang KK, Lutzke LS, et al. Combined endoscopic mucosal resection and photodynamic therapy for esophageal neoplasia within Barrett's esophagus. Gastrointest Endosc 2001;54(6):682–8.
25. Schnell TG, Sontag SJ, Chejfec G, et al. Long-term nonsurgical management of Barrett's esophagus with high-grade dysplasia. Gastroenterology 2001;120(7):1607–19.
26. Reid BJ, Levine DS, Longton G, et al. Predictors of progression to cancer in Barrett's esophagus: baseline histology and flow cytometry identify low- and high-risk patient subsets. Am J Gastroenterol 2000;95(7):1669–76.
27. Weston AP, Sharma P. Neodymium:yttrium-aluminum garnet contact laser ablation of Barrett's high grade dysplasia and early adenocarcinoma. Am J Gastroenterol 2002;97(12):2998–3006.
28. Hameeteman W, Tytgat GN, Houthoff HJ, et al. Barrett's esophagus: development of dysplasia and adenocarcinoma. Gastroenterology 1989;96(5 Pt 1):1249–56.
29. Zaninotto G, Minnei F, Guirroli E, et al. The Veneto Region's Barrett's Oesophagus Registry: aims, methods, preliminary results. Dig Liver Dis 2007;39(1):18–25.
30. Tokar JL, Haluszka O, Weinberg DS. Endoscopic therapy of dysplasia and early-stage cancers of the esophagus. Semin Radiat Oncol 2007;17(1):10–21.
31. Dougherty TJ. An update on photodynamic therapy applications. J Clin Laser Med Surg 2002;20(1):3–7.
32. Dougherty TJ, Gomer CJ, Henderson BW, et al. Photodynamic therapy. J Natl Cancer Inst 1998;90(12):889–905.
33. Ackroyd R, Kelty C, Brown N, et al. The history of photodetection and photodynamic therapy. Photochem Photobiol 2001;74(5):656–69.
34. Bown SG, Rogowska AZ. New photosensitizers for photodynamic therapy in gastroenterology. Can J Gastroenterol 1999;13(5):389–92.

35. Bellnier DA, Greco WR, Nava H, et al. Mild skin photosensitivity in cancer patients following injection of Photochlor (2-[1-hexyloxyethyl]-2-devinyl pyro-pheophorbide-a; HPPH) for photodynamic therapy. Cancer Chemother Pharmacol 2006;57(1):40–5.
36. Overholt B, Panjehpour M, Tefftellar E, et al. Photodynamic therapy for treatment of early adenocarcinoma in Barrett's esophagus. Gastrointest Endosc 1993; 39(1):73–6.
37. Overholt BF, Panjehpour M, Haydek JM. Photodynamic therapy for Barrett's esophagus: follow-up in 100 patients. Gastrointest Endosc 1999; 49(1):1–7.
38. Wang KK, Kim JY. Photodynamic therapy in Barrett's esophagus. Gastrointest Endosc Clin N Am 2003;13(3):483–9, vii.
39. Wolfsen HC, Woodward TA, Raimondo M. Photodynamic therapy for dysplastic Barrett esophagus and early esophageal adenocarcinoma. Mayo Clin Proc 2002;77(11):1176–81.
40. Wolfsen HC, Hemminger LL, Wallace MB, et al. Clinical experience of patients undergoing photodynamic therapy for Barrett's dysplasia or cancer. Aliment Pharmacol Ther 2004;20(10):1125–31.
41. Wang KK, Wong Kee Song LM, Buttar NS, et al. Barrett's esophagus after photodynamic therapy: risk of cancer development during long term follow up [abstract]. Gastroenterology 2004;126(Suppl 2):A50.
42. Wolfsen HC, Hemminger LL. Photodynamic therapy for dysplastic Barrett's esophagus and mucosal adenocarcinoma [abstract]. Gastrointest Endosc 2004;59(5):AB251.
43. Ukleja A, Scolapio JS, Wolfsen HC. Nutritional consequences following photodynamic therapy. Gastrotenterology 1999;116(4 Part 2):A582.
44. Nijhawan PK, Wang KK. Endoscopic mucosal resection for lesions with endoscopic features suggestive of malignancy and high-grade dysplasia within Barrett's esophagus. Gastrointest Endosc 2000;52(3):328–32.
45. Panjehpour M, Overholt BF, Haydek JM, et al. Results of photodynamic therapy for ablation of dysplasia and early cancer in Barrett's esophagus and effect of oral steroids on stricture formation. Am J Gastroenterol 2000; 95(9):2177–84.
46. Pacifico RJ, Wang KK, Wong Kee Song LM, et al. Combined endoscopic mucosal resection and photodynamic therapy versus esophagectomy for management of early adenocarcinoma in Barrett's esophagus. Clin Gastroenterol Hepatol 2003;1(4):252–7.
47. Prasad GA, Wang KK, Buttar NS, et al. Long-term survival following endoscopic and surgical treatment of high-grade dysplasia in Barrett's esophagus. Gastroenterology 2007;132(4):1226–33.
48. Foroulis CN, Thorpe JA. Photodynamic therapy (PDT) in Barrett's esophagus with dysplasia or early cancer. Eur J Cardiothorac Surg 2006;29(1):30–4.
49. Keeley SB, Pennathur A, Gooding W, et al. Photodynamic therapy with curative intent for Barrett's esophagus with high grade dysplasia and superficial esophageal cancer. Ann Surg Oncol 2007;14(8):2406–10.
50. Hemminger LL, Wolfsen HC. Photodynamic therapy for Barrett's esophagus and high grade dysplasia: results of a patient satisfaction survey. Gastroenterol Nurs 2002;25(4):139–41.
51. Hur C, Nishioka NS, Gazelle GS. Cost-effectiveness of photodynamic therapy for treatment of Barrett's esophagus with high grade dysplasia. Dig Dis Sci 2003; 48(7):1273–83.

52. Wolfsen HC, Hemminger LL, DeVault KR. Barrett's dysplasia and mucosal carcinoma patients referred for photodynamic therapy – do they come from surveillance programs? [abstract]. Gastrointest Endosc 2004;59(5):AB265.

53. Bronner MP, Overholt BF, Taylor SL, et al. Squamous overgrowth is not a safety concern for photodynamic therapy for Barrett's esophagus with high-grade dysplasia. Gastroenterology 2009;136(1):56–64, quiz 351–2.

54. Yachimski P, Puricelli WP, Nishioka NS. Patient predictors of esophageal stricture development after photodynamic therapy. Clin Gastroenterol Hepatol 2008;6(3): 302–8.

55. Andrejevic-Blant S, Hadjur C, Ballini JP, et al. Photodynamic therapy of early squamous cell carcinoma with tetra(m-hydroxyphenyl)chlorin: optimal drug-light interval. Br J Cancer 1997;76(8):1021–8.

56. Andrejevic-Blant S, Grosjean P, Ballini JP, et al. Localization of tetra(m-hydroxyphenyl)chlorin (Foscan) in human healthy tissues and squamous cell carcinomas of the upper aero-digestive tract, the esophagus and the bronchi: a fluorescence microscopy study. J Photochem Photobiol B 2001;61(1–2):1–9.

57. Gossner L, May A, Sroka R, et al. A new long-range through-the-scope balloon applicator for photodynamic therapy in the esophagus and cardia. Endoscopy 1999;31(5):370–6.

58. Gossner L, May A, Sroka R, et al. Photodynamic destruction of high grade dysplasia and early carcinoma of the esophagus after the oral administration of 5-aminolevulinic acid. Cancer 1999;86(10):1921–8.

59. Gossner L, Stolte M, Sroka R, et al. Photodynamic ablation of high-grade dysplasia and early cancer in Barrett's esophagus by means of 5-aminolevulinic acid. Gastroenterology 1998;114(3):448–55.

60. Javaid B, Watt P, Krasner N. Photodynamic therapy (PDT) for oesophageal dysplasia and early carcinoma with mTHPC (m-tetrahydroxyphenyl chlorin): a preliminary study. Lasers Med Sci 2002;17(1):51–6.

61. Etienne J, Dorme N, Bourg-Heckly G, et al. Photodynamic therapy with green light and m-tetrahydroxyphenyl chlorin for intramucosal adenocarcinoma and high-grade dysplasia in Barrett's esophagus. Gastrointest Endosc 2004;59(7):880–9.

62. Lovat LB, Jamieson NF, Novelli MR, et al. Photodynamic therapy with m-tetrahydroxyphenyl chlorin for high-grade dysplasia and early cancer in Barrett's columnar lined esophagus. Gastrointest Endosc 2005;62(4):617–23.

63. Bedwell J, MacRobert AJ, Phillips D, et al. Fluorescence distribution and photodynamic effect of ALA-induced PP IX in the DMH rat colonic tumour model. Br J Cancer 1992;65(6):818–24.

64. Kennedy JC, Pottier RH. Endogenous protoporphyrin IX, a clinically useful photosensitizer for photodynamic therapy. J Photochem Photobiol B 1992; 14(4):275–92.

65. Peng Q, Berg K, Moan J, et al. 5-Aminolevulinic acid-based photodynamic therapy: principles and experimental research. Photochem Photobiol 1997; 65(2):235–51.

66. Webber J, Kessel D, Fromm D. Side effects and photosensitization of human tissues after aminolevulinic acid. J Surg Res 1997;68(1):31–7.

67. Ackroyd R, Brown NJ, Davis MF, et al. Photodynamic therapy for dysplastic Barrett's oesophagus: a prospective, double blind, randomised, placebo controlled trial. Gut 2000;47(5):612–7.

68. Ackroyd R, Brown NJ, Davis MF, et al. Aminolevulinic acid-induced photodynamic therapy: safe and effective ablation of dysplasia in Barrett's esophagus. Dis Esophagus 2000;13(1):18–22.

69. Barr H, Shepherd NA, Dix A, et al. Eradication of high-grade dysplasia in columnar-lined (Barrett's) oesophagus by photodynamic therapy with endogenously generated protoporphyrin IX. Lancet 1996;348(9027):584–5.
70. Orth K, Stanescu A, Ruck A, et al. [Photodynamic ablation and argon-plasma coagulation of premalignant and early-stage malignant lesions of the oesophagus–an alternative to surgery?]. Chirurg 1999;70(4):431–8 [in German].
71. Pech O, Gossner L, May A, et al. Long term results of PDT for early neoplasia in Barrett's esophagus. Gastrointest Endosc 2005;62(1):24–30.
72. Guelrud M, Herrera I, Essenfeld H, et al. Enhanced magnification endoscopy: a new technique to identify specialized intestinal metaplasia in Barrett's esophagus. Gastrointest Endosc 2001;53(6):559–65.
73. Behrens A, May A, Gossner L, et al. Curative treatment for high-grade intraepithelial neoplasia in Barrett's esophagus. Endoscopy 2005;37(10):999–1005.
74. May A, Gossner L, Pech O, et al. Intraepithelial high-grade neoplasia and early adenocarcinoma in short-segment Barrett's esophagus (SSBE): curative treatment using local endoscopic treatment techniques. Endoscopy 2002;34(8):604–10.
75. Sylantiev C, Schoenfeld N, Mamet R, et al. Acute neuropathy mimicking porphyria induced by aminolevulinic acid during photodynamic therapy. Muscle Nerve 2005;31(3):390–3.
76. Siersema PD. Photodynamic therapy for Barrett's esophagus: not yet ready for the premier league of endoscopic interventions. Gastrointest Endosc 2005; 62(4):503–7.
77. Ortner MA, Zumbusch K, Liebetruth J, et al. Is topical delta-aminolevulinic acid adequate for photodynamic therapy in Barrett's esophagus? A pilot study. Endoscopy 2002;34(8):611–6.
78. Ragunath K, Krasner N, Raman VS, et al. Endoscopic ablation of dysplastic Barrett's oesophagus comparing argon plasma coagulation and photodynamic therapy: a randomized prospective trial assessing efficacy and cost-effectiveness. Scand J Gastroenterol 2005;40(7):750–8.
79. Kelty CJ, Ackroyd R, Brown NJ, et al. Comparison of high- vs low-dose 5-aminolevulinic acid for photodynamic therapy of Barrett's esophagus. Surg Endosc 2004;18(3):452–8.
80. Kelty CJ, Ackroyd R, Brown NJ, et al. Endoscopic ablation of Barrett's oesophagus: a randomized-controlled trial of photodynamic therapy vs. argon plasma coagulation. Aliment Pharmacol Ther 2004;20(11–12):1289–96.
81. Hage M, Siersema PD, van Dekken H, et al. 5-Aminolevulinic acid photodynamic therapy versus argon plasma coagulation for ablation of Barrett's oesophagus: a randomised trial. Gut 2004;53(6):785–90.
82. Peters F, Kara M, Rosmolen W, et al. Poor results of 5-aminolevulinic acid-photodynamic therapy for residual high-grade dysplasia and early cancer in Barrett esophagus after endoscopic resection. Endoscopy 2005;37(5):418–24.
83. Mackenzie G, Selvasekar C, Jamieson N, et al. Low incidence of esophageal adenocarcinoma following optimal regimen of ALA PDT for high grade dysplasia in Barrett's esophagus [abstract]. Gastrointest Endosc 2007;65(5):AB132.
84. Boere IA, Robinson DJ, de Bruijn HS, et al. Monitoring in situ dosimetry and protoporphyrin IX fluorescence photobleaching in the normal rat esophagus during 5-aminolevulinic acid photodynamic therapy. Photochem Photobiol 2003;78(3):271–7.
85. Cheung R, Solonenko M, Busch TM, et al. Correlation of in vivo photosensitizer fluorescence and photodynamic-therapy-induced depth of necrosis in a murine tumor model. J Biomed Opt 2003;8(2):248–52.

86. Radu A, Conde R, Fontolliet C, et al. Mucosal ablation with photodynamic therapy in the esophagus: optimization of light dosimetry in the sheep model. Gastrointest Endosc 2003;57(7):897–905.
87. Panjehpour M, Overholt BF, Phan MN, et al. Optimization of light dosimetry for photodynamic therapy of Barrett's esophagus: efficacy vs. incidence of stricture after treatment. Gastrointest Endosc 2005;61(1):13–8.
88. Gill KR, Wolfsen HC, Preyer NW, et al. Pilot study on light dosimetry variables for photodynamic therapy of Barrett's esophagus with high-grade dysplasia. Clin Cancer Res 2009;15(5):1830–6.
89. van den Bergh H. On the evolution of some endoscopic light delivery systems for photodynamic therapy. Endoscopy 1998;30(4):392–407.
90. Panjehpour M, Overholt BF, Haydek JM. Light sources and delivery devices for photodynamic therapy in the gastrointestinal tract. Gastrointest Endosc Clin N Am 2000;10(3):513–32.
91. Overholt BF, Panjehpour M, DeNovo RC, et al. Balloon photodynamic therapy of esophageal cancer: effect of increasing balloon size. Lasers Surg Med 1996; 18(3):248–52.
92. Prasad GA, Wang KK, Buttar NS, et al. Predictors of stricture formation after photodynamic therapy for high-grade dysplasia in Barrett's esophagus. Gastrointest Endosc 2007;65(1):60–6.
93. Stepinac T, Grosjean P, Woodtli A, et al. Optimization of the diameter of a radial irradiation device for photodynamic therapy in the esophagus. Endoscopy 2002; 34(5):411–5.
94. Braichotte DR, Savary JF, Monnier P, et al. Optimizing light dosimetry in photodynamic therapy of early stage carcinomas of the esophagus using fluorescence spectroscopy. Lasers Surg Med 1996;19(3):340–6.
95. Zellweger M, Grosjean P, Monnier P, et al. Stability of the fluorescence measurement of Foscan in the normal human oral cavity as an indicator of its content in early cancers of the esophagus and the bronchi. Photochem Photobiol 1999; 69(5):605–10.
96. Standish BA, Yang VX, Munce NR, et al. Doppler optical coherence tomography monitoring of microvascular tissue response during photodynamic therapy in an animal model of Barrett's esophagus. Gastrointest Endosc 2007;66(2):326–33.
97. Wong DJ, Paulson TG, Prevo LJ, et al. p16(INK4a) lesions are common, early abnormalities that undergo clonal expansion in Barrett's metaplastic epithelium. Cancer Res 2001;61(22):8284–9.
98. Prevo LJ, Sanchez CA, Galipeau PC, et al. p53-mutant clones and field effects in Barrett's esophagus. Cancer Res 1999;59(19):4784–7.
99. Prasad GA, Wang KK, Halling KC, et al. Correlation of histology with biomarker status after photodynamic therapy in Barrett esophagus. Cancer 2008;113(3): 470–6.
100. Hornick JL, Mino-Kenudson M, Lauwers GY, et al. Buried Barrett's epithelium following photodynamic therapy shows reduced crypt proliferation and absence of DNA content abnormalities. Am J Gastroenterol 2008;103(1):38–47.
101. Panjehpour M, Coppola D, Overholt BF, et al. Photodynamic therapy of Barrett's esophagus: ablation of Barrett's mucosa and reduction in p53 protein expression after treatment. Anticancer Res 2008;28(1B):485–9.
102. Ginsberg GG, Furth EE, Ginsberg J, et al. Multi-modal endoluminal eradication therapy for specialized intestinal metaplasia of the esophagus and the

esophagogastric junction with high-grade dysplasia and/or intramucosal carcinoma. Gastrointest Endosc Clin N Am 2007;65(5):AB154.

103. Shaheen NJ, Sharma P, Overholt BF, et al. Radiofrequency ablation in Barrett's esophagus with dysplasia. N Engl J Med 2009;360(22):2277–88.

104. Kahaleh M, Van Laethem JL, Nagy N, et al. Long-term follow-up and factors predictive of recurrence in Barrett's esophagus treated by argon plasma coagulation and acid suppression. Endoscopy 2002;34(12):950–5.

105. Shaheen NJ, Inadomi JM, Overholt BF, et al. What is the best management strategy for high grade dysplasia in Barrett's oesophagus? A cost effectiveness analysis. Gut 2004;53(12):1736–44.

106. Tan WC, Fulljames C, Stone N, et al. Photodynamic therapy using 5-aminolaevulinic acid for oesophageal adenocarcinoma associated with Barrett's metaplasia. J Photochem Photobiol B 1999;53(1–3):75–80.

107. Mackenzie GD, Jamieson NF, Novelli MR, et al. How light dosimetry influences the efficacy of photodynamic therapy with 5-aminolaevulinic acid for ablation of high-grade dysplasia in Barrett's esophagus. Lasers Med Sci 2008;23(2): 203–10.

108. Ackroyd R, Kelty CJ, Brown NJ, et al. Eradication of dysplastic Barrett's oesophagus using photodynamic therapy: long-term follow-up. Endoscopy 2003;35(6): 496–501.

Endoscopic Therapy Using Radiofrequency Ablation for Esophageal Dysplasia and Carcinoma in Barrett's Esophagus

Frederike G.I. van Vilsteren, MD, Jacques J.G.H.M. Bergman, MD, PhD *

KEYWORDS

- Esophagus • Barrett • Radiofrequency ablation
- Endoscopic resection • Endoscopy • Dysplasia • Neoplasia

Barrett's esophagus (BE) is a premalignant condition in which the normal squamous cell lining of the esophagus is replaced by columnar epithelium containing specialized intestinal metaplasia (IM), defined by the presence of goblet cells.[1] The most important risk factor for BE is chronic gastroesophageal reflux disease (GERD). BE is found in approximately 10% of patients undergoing endoscopy for chronic GERD symptoms[2] and therefore it is hypothesized that the transition from squamous mucosa into mucus-secreting columnar epithelium is an adaptation of esophageal mucosa caused by the erosive effect of the refluxate. Via a gradual process from no dysplasia to low-grade (LGD) and high-grade dysplasia (HGD), BE can develop into adenocarcinoma.[3-5] The estimated annual incidence of adenocarcinoma in BE is 0.5%.[6-8] When esophageal cancer enters a symptomatic stage, disease is usually locally advanced and has a poor prognosis with a 5-year survival of approximately 20%.[9-11] For patients with HGD or early cancer, previously surgical resection was the gold standard. Surgical esophagectomy is, however, associated with a mortality rate of 3% to 5% and serious complications occur in 40% to 50% of patients.[12-14] In the subset of patients with "early neoplasia", defined as HGD or intramucosal cancer, lymph node involvement is rare: 0% for HGD and up to 2% for intramucosal cancer.[15,16] As a result,

Disclosures: J.J.G.H.M.B. has received grants and materials for research support from the following companies: AstraZeneca (Zoetermeer, Netherlands), BÂRRX (Sunnyvale, CA), Olympus Endoscopy (Hamburg, Germany; Tokyo, Japan), and Cook Medical (Limerick, Ireland).
Department of Gastroenterology and Hepatology, Academic Medical Center, University of Amsterdam, Meibergdreef 9, 1105 AZ, Amsterdam, The Netherlands
* Corresponding author.
E-mail address: j.j.bergman@amc.uva.nl (J.J.G.H.M. Bergman).

Gastrointest Endoscopy Clin N Am 20 (2010) 55–74
doi:10.1016/j.giec.2009.07.007
1052-5157/09/$ – see front matter © 2010 Elsevier Inc. All rights reserved.

endoscopic treatment of early neoplastic lesions is a viable alternative to surgery for these patients.

ENDOSCOPIC TREATMENT MODALITIES

Endoscopic treatment comprises endoscopic resection (ER) and endoscopic ablation techniques. The most important advantage of ER above ablation therapy is that ER results in a resection specimen for histopathological assessment, contributing to optimal staging and patient selection. Although ER is a safe and effective treatment modality, with 5-year disease-specific survival of 95%,[17] metachronous lesions arising in the residual BE segment can be found after ER in 30% of patients.[18]

To eliminate the malignant potential after ER, eradication of the residual BE epithelium is advocated. To accomplish this, treatment protocols combining ER and ablation therapy have been developed. Photodynamic therapy (PDT) using amino levulinic acid (ALA) or porfimer sodium (Ps) and argon plasma coagulation (APC) are ablation techniques that have been administered for this purpose, but both techniques have disappointingly high rates of recurrent early neoplasia and residual IM.[19,20] In both PDT and APC, ablation depth is not controlled and may vary, resulting in residual BE that still carries preexistent oncogenetic abnormalities.[21,22] Sometimes residual BE glands become hidden underneath neosquamous epithelium (ie, "buried Barrett's glands"), and some fear that these may progress to dysplasia or cancer without being detected endoscopically.[23,24] Another complication from porfimer sodium (Ps-PDT) and APC is a high stenosis rate, which may be a result of submucosal scarring owing to uncontrolled ablation depth.[19,20] Finally, Ps-PDT is associated with significant photosensitivity for a period of up to 6 weeks after treatment.[25]

An alternative to ablation therapy is the complete removal of the BE by radical endoscopic resection (RER), generally performed in multiple treatment sessions. Small-sized single-center studies have reported low recurrence rates of early neoplasia after RER varying from 0% to 9% after up to 28 months of follow-up, and newly formed squamous epithelium after RER has been shown free of oncogenetic abnormalities. However, symptomatic stenosis develops in up to 56% of patients, requiring multiple dilations sessions.[26-30]

The latest treatment modality for complete removal of BE is radiofrequency ablation (RFA). This novel ablation technique has shown excellent results for selected patients with nondysplastic BE, LGD, and HGD with or without prior ER with a follow-up of almost 2 years. Regarding the safety and efficacy profile, RFA compares favorably to other ablation techniques such as PDT and APC.[31,32]

RADIOFREQUENCY ABLATION: THE HALO SYSTEM

The HALO system (BÂRRX Medical, Sunnyvale, CA) (**Fig. 1**) for RFA is designed to control tissue penetration depth of the RF energy of 0.5 mm, thereby realizing a uniform ablation depth that is operator independent, owing to the use of bipolar electrodes and the automated delivery of a preset amount of RF energy. The HALO system consists of a circumferential and a focal ablation device for stepwise ablation of the BE epithelium. For larger areas of BE, circumferential ablation is performed using the HALO^{360}-device, a balloon-based catheter with spindle-shaped electrodes covering a length of 3 mm. The HALO^{360}-balloon is available in several diameters: 18, 22, 25, 28, 31, and 34 mm. Ablation using the HALO^{360}-balloon is performed with an energy density of 12 J/cm^2 and 40 Watt/cm^2. For focal ablation of residual BE epithelium, the endoscope-mounted HALO^{90}-device is developed. The HALO^{90}-device is equipped with an articulating surface containing an electrode array (13 mm wide × 20 mm

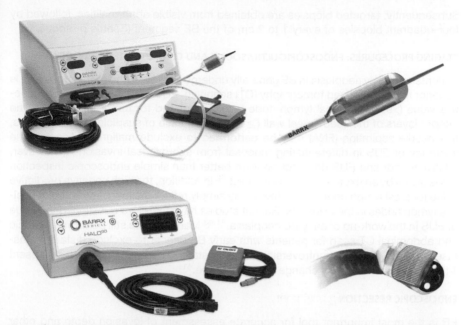

Fig. 1. The HALO system for stepwise circumferential and focal radiofrequency ablation (RFA). (*Upper left*) The HALO^{360} generator with integrated pressure:volume system, used to inflate the sizing and ablation catheters, to calculate esophageal inner diameter, and to deliver radiofrequency energy to the ablation catheter. (*Upper right*) The HALO^{360+} ablation catheter. (*Lower left*) The HALO^{90} energy generator for delivery of radiofrequency energy. (*Lower right*) The HALO^{90} catheter fitted on the tip of an endoscope, without impairing the endoscopic view or function. (*Reproduced from* www.endosurgery.eu; with permission. *Courtesy of* ER and RFA Training Program, Amsterdam, The Netherlands; with permission.)

long) to target small areas of BE with an energy density of 15 J/cm^2 and a power of 40 W/cm^2.

PATIENT SELECTION FOR ENDOSCOPIC MANAGEMENT OF EARLY NEOPLASIA

To correctly select the subgroup of patients suitable for RFA treatment, a thorough work-up and staging protocol is mandatory. In general, patients with early neoplasia in BE are considered potential candidates for endoscopic treatment when the lesion is limited in size (<2 cm), there are no signs of deep submucosal invasion, and no suspicious lymph nodes are found on endoscopic ultrasound (EUS). The tumor characteristics are of importance in staging, as the risk for lymph node involvement increases with increasing infiltration depth, poor differentiation grade, and lymphatic/vascular-invasive tumor growth.[11,16,33,34]

IMAGING ENDOSCOPY

Optimal endoscopic treatment of patients with early BE neoplasia starts with at least one high-resolution endoscopy by an experienced endoscopist. During inspection, visible abnormalities are classified according to the Paris classification.[35,36] The Prague-CM-classification is used to describe the BE segment, including the length of the circumferential segment (C), and the maximal extent of the BE segment (M).[37]

Subsequently, targeted biopsies are obtained from visible abnormalities, followed by four-quadrant biopsies of every 1 to 2 cm of the BE segment (Seattle protocol).[38]

STAGING PROCEDURES: ENDOSCOPIC ULTRASOUND AND COMPUTERIZED TOMOGRAPHY

Patients with early neoplasia in BE generally undergo EUS for T and N staging, which is superior to computerized tomography (CT) scanning. EUS has a high negative predictive value (>95%) for local lymph node involvement and for tumor infiltration in the deeper layers of the esophageal wall ($\geq$ T2).[39–41] In case of suspicious lymph nodes, fine-needle aspiration (FNA) may be performed to exclude malignant disease. The accuracy of EUS in differentiating mucosal from submucosal invasion is, however, relatively poor and EUS does not perform better than simple endoscopic inspection of the lesion by an experienced endoscopist.[42] In addition, the high negative predictive value for local lymph node involvement may simply reflect the low prevalence of positive lymph nodes in these lesions. Recent studies have therefore questioned the value of EUS in the work-up of early BE neoplasia.[41,43] Many centers still perform a thoracic and abdominal CT scan for patients with early BE cancer to exclude distant metastases. This is however controversial, as the distant metastases are virtually absent T1 lesions and thus rarely change the TNM stage.[41]

ENDOSCOPIC RESECTION

ER is the most important tool for accurate assessment of invasion depth and other histologic tumor characteristics (differentiation grade, lymphatic invasion). ER therefore serves both a diagnostic as well as therapeutic purpose. Diagnostic in the sense that it correctly identifies patients with submucosal invasion, poor differentiation grade, and/or lymphatic invasion; therapeutic in the sense that it allows removal of all visible (ie, nonflat mucosa) lesions thus rendering the remaining BE segment flat and thereby suitable for RFA. The two most widely used techniques are the ER-cap technique and the Multi Band Mucosectomy (MBM) technique; both are safe and effective for "en bloc" as well as "piecemeal" resections.[44,45]

HISTOPATHOLOGICAL ASSESSMENT

For the histopathological evaluation of biopsies or resection specimens, the revised Vienna classification is used.[46,47] After ER, patients are suitable candidates for further endoscopic management, if the resection specimen shows negative vertical resection margins, no submucosal tumor infiltration, well- or moderate tumor differentiation (G1-G2), and no lymphatic/vascular invasion. Because early BE neoplasia is not frequently encountered by community pathologists, it is imperative that the histopathological evaluation is performed by a pathologist with experience in this field.

WORK-UP FOR RADIOFREQUENCY ABLATION

Before RFA, all carcinoma has to be completely removed and the epithelium should be endoscopically flat. This is required because the HALO electrodes for RFA are designed to perform controlled superficial ablation of 0.5 mm and are unlikely to be effective for neoplasia in thickened mucosa. Most RFA studies have excluded patients with invasive cancer at baseline and biopsies should therefore be taken from the residual BE segment after ER. Also, in most studies, an additional endoscopy was performed 4 to 6 weeks after the ER session to exclude visible abnormalities and to obtain four quadrant biopsies from the BE segment to rule out invasive cancer. At that time, however, the edges of the ER scar may be slightly elevated because of reactive changes, which may be misinterpreted as visible abnormalities. The most optimal time to exclude the presence of residual visible abnormalities and to obtain biopsies from the residual BE is thus immediately after the ER in the same session.

When the mucosa is flat and biopsies contain no invasive cancer, the patient is scheduled for an RFA session 6 to 8 weeks after ER.

PERFORMING CIRCUMFERENTIAL ABLATION: USE OF THE HALO³⁶⁰-DEVICE

RFA procedures can be performed on an outpatient basis using conscious sedation. At the initial ablation session, the extent of the BE segment determines if the patient will be treated with the HALO³⁶⁰-balloon or with the focal HALO⁹⁰-device. When the circumferential BE segment is smaller than 2 cm in length, or consists only of tongues and/or islands smaller than 2 cm, the patient can be primarily treated with focal ablation.[48,49] Most frequently, patients initially require circumferential ablation, which involves the following steps:

(1) Inspection and recording of esophageal landmarks

Before ablation, the esophagus is inspected to confirm the flat aspect of the mucosa, to exclude the presence of esophagitis, and to record the esophageal landmarks according to the Prague CM classification.[35] After inspection, the esophagus wall is sprayed with 20 mL of acetylcysteine (1%, watery solution) to remove excessive mucus, followed by flushing with plain water.

(2) Sizing procedure (**Fig. 2**).

Subsequently, the esophageal inner diameter (EID) is measured, to select an appropriate ablation balloon, allowing for optimal contact between electrode and esophageal wall without applying too much pressure. A 4-cm long noncompliant sizing balloon-catheter is connected to the generator with an interposed air filter. After calibration, the sizing balloon is inserted over a 0.035-in guide wire (Amplatz extra stiff, Cook Endoscopy, Limerick, Ireland), omitting lubricant jelly for introduction, exclusively using water.

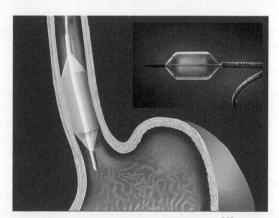

Fig. 2. The sizing procedure using the HALO system. The HALO³⁶⁰ generator with integrated pressure:volume system automatically inflates and deflates the sizing balloon, to calculate esophageal inner diameter. The esophageal inner diameter is measured for each centimeter of the Barrett's segment from proximal to distal, to adequately select the size of the ablation balloon. (*Reproduced from* www.endosurgery.eu; with permission. *Courtesy of* ER and RFA Training Program, Amsterdam, The Netherlands; with permission.)

Sizing is performed for every centimeter of the BE segment, starting 5 cm above the most proximal extent of the BE, using the centimeter scale on the catheter shaft for reference (discordant to the centimeter scale of the endoscope). For sizing, the balloon is automatically inflated to 4 psi (0.28 atm) after pressing a foot switch, and automatically deflated after measurement. The mean EID over 4 cm is then calculated with a pressure-volume algorithm and displayed on the generator. When a strong increase in the measured EID indicates that the sizing balloon has reached the hiatal hernia or stomach, the sizing balloon is removed, leaving the guide wire in place.

(3) Selection of the appropriate ablation balloon:

The smallest measured EID defines the appropriate balloon diameter. For patients without prior ER, the recommended balloon diameter is the one closest to the smallest measurement (eg, if the smallest EID is 24 mm, a 25-mm ablation balloon is chosen; if the EID is 23 mm, the 22-mm ablation balloon is appropriate). For patients with a prior ER or stenosis, a balloon that is two sizes smaller than the smallest measurement has to be selected, to reduce the risk for laceration (eg, if the smallest EID is 26 mm, a 22-mm ablation balloon should be used). When a suitable ablation balloon size has been selected, the ablation balloon catheter is inserted over the guide wire followed by introduction of the endoscope alongside for visualization of the ablation procedure.

(4) First ablation pass (**Fig. 3**).

For ablation with the HALO^{360}-device, the surface is treated with two energy deliveries of 12 J/cm^2 with cleaning of the ablation zone in between ablation passes, referred to as the "double" regimen. Ablation is performed from proximal to distal starting 1 cm above the most proximal extent of the BE segment, allowing for a maximal overlap of 0.5 to 1.0 cm. Before ablation, the endoscope and ablation catheter are fixed to the bite block to avoid dislocation of the balloon by inflation. After inflation of the ablation balloon, as initiated by the endoscopist using the foot switch, suctioning is applied for optimal contact between electrode and epithelium. Next, the endoscopist starts the ablation, resulting in RF energy delivery and automatic deflation of the balloon. Ablation renders the BE epithelium white, which helps in identifying the subsequent BE zone when advancing the deflated ablation balloon distally. After ablation of the complete BE segment, the ablation balloon, guide wire, and endoscope are removed simultaneously.

(5) Cleaning procedure:

After the first ablation pass, the coagulum is cleaned off the ablation surface and the balloon electrode before the second ablation pass. Cleaning in between the ablation passes has been shown to increase the efficacy of the initial ablation session from 90% to 95%.[50–52] Debris is gently pushed off the ablated area using the rim of the small flexible cap (eg, HALO cap; BÂRRX Medical or Olympus zoom cap, MB0-046; Olympus, Tokyo, Japan), mounted on the tip of the endoscope, followed by forcefully spraying with plain water using a spraying catheter (eg, Olympus PV-5-1; Olympus) and a high-pressure pistol (eg, Alliance; Boston Scientific, Limerick, Ireland). Cleaning of the balloon electrode is performed outside the patient using plain water and a gauze, being careful to wipe "with the grain" of the electrode array.

(6) Second ablation pass:

After the cleaning procedure, the guide wire and ablation balloon are reinserted followed by the endoscope, as before, and a second ablation pass is performed from

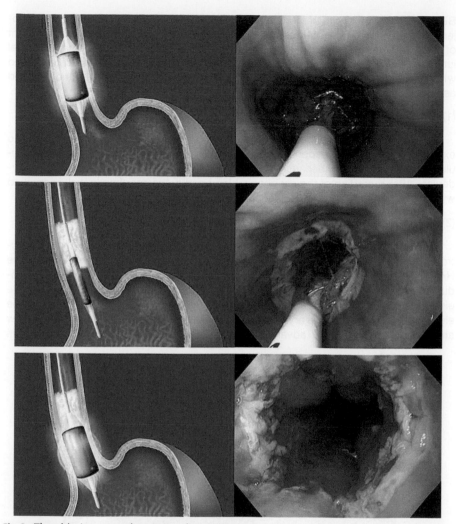

Fig. 3. The ablation procedure using the HALO system. Ablation is performed from proximal to distal starting 1 cm above the most proximal extent of the Barrett's segment. (*Upper*) The ablation balloon is inflated and ablation is performed upon activation using the foot switch. (*Middle*) After ablation, the Barrett's epithelium shows a white debris, which helps identifying the subsequent BE zone when advancing the deflated ablation balloon distally. (*Lower*) Subsequent ablations are performed allowing for a maximal overlap of 0.5 to 1.0 cm, until the complete Barrett's segment has been ablated. (*Reproduced from* www. endosurgery.eu; with permission. *Courtesy of* ER and RFA Training Program, Amsterdam, The Netherlands; with permission.)

proximal to distal, resulting in a brownish discoloration of the previously ablated BE epithelium.

PERFORMING FOCAL ABLATION: USE OF THE HALO⁹⁰-DEVICE

Two to 3 months after initial ablation, upper endoscopy with narrow band imaging (NBI) is performed to assess BE regression. Patients with a residual circumferential

BE segment with a length of more than 2 cm and/or multiple isles or tongues are subjected to a second circumferential ablation session. In case the circumferential extent of residual BE is less than 2 cm in length, and/or there is an irregular gastroesophageal junction, and/or tongues and islands are smaller than 2 cm in size, this can be treated with the HALO^{90}-device for focal ablation. The focal ablation procedure is performed as follows:

(1) Inspection and recording of esophageal landmarks:

Again the esophagus is inspected to confirm the flat aspect of the mucosa and to exclude the presence of esophagitis. Additionally, the presence of a Zenker's diverticulum has to be excluded because this may complicate the introduction of the HALO^{90}-device. After recording of the esophageal landmarks, the esophagus wall is sprayed with acetylcysteine (1%) and flushed with plain water.

(2) Introduction of the HALO^{90}-catheter (**Fig. 4**).

The HALO^{90}-catheter is attached to the distal end of the endoscope, and the electrode cap placed at the 12 o'clock position in the endoscopic field of view. The HALO^{90}-device is inserted without using lubricant jelly but only water to facilitate introduction. After advancing the HALO^{90}-electrode surface over the tongue, the top of the electrode is deflected downwards when the laryngeal cavity is visualized, to allow the electrode to pass behind the arytenoids. Subsequently, the patient is asked to swallow and the catheter is gently advanced. When introduction of the HALO^{90}-device is

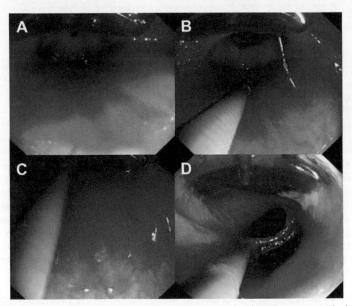

Fig. 4. (*A*) The leading edge of the HALO cap is visible proximal to the arytenoids. (*B*) A biopsy forceps is blindly advanced behind the arytenoids into the proximal esophagus. (*C*) The endoscope is angulated downward, causing the leading edge of the HALO cap to touch the shaft of the biopsy forceps. (*D*) After gently advancing the endoscope, using the biopsy forceps for guidance, the proximal esophagus is entered. (*Reproduced from* www.endosurgery.eu; with permission. *Courtesy of* ER and RFA Training Program, Amsterdam, The Netherlands; with permission.)

difficult, a biopsy forceps or the spraying catheter can be used to guide the instrument into the esophagus. With the endoscope in the hypopharynx, the forceps is advanced under direct view dorsal to the arytenoids deep into the esophagus. The endoscope is angled down so that the leading edge of the HALO^{90}-device can slide over the forceps while the endoscope is gently advanced. Other techniques for difficult intubations include Savary dilation (45 Fr) followed by leaving the guide wire in place to facilitate passage of the HALO^{90}-device.

(3) First ablation pass (**Fig. 5**).

In the esophagus, the HALO^{90}-electrode surface is positioned against the wall at the target area. Optimal contact between electrode and esophageal wall is obtained by upward deflection of the tip of the endoscope. For ablation with the HALO^{90}-device, the "double-double" regimen is administered. Ablation is initiated by the endoscopist using the foot switch, and after an area has been treated with an energy delivery of 15 J/cm^2, a second energy delivery of 15 J/cm^2 is realized immediately after the first, while keeping the electrode in place. After treatment of the residual BE areas, the Z-line is ablated by circumferentially applying the HALO^{90}-device, to eliminate the potential of a small rim of residual BE epithelium at the Z-line, which is endoscopically indistinguishable from gastric epithelium.

(4) Cleaning procedure:

After the first ablation pass, debris is cleaned off the ablated area by carefully pushing with the HALO^{90}-electrode in the proximal-to-distal direction, combined

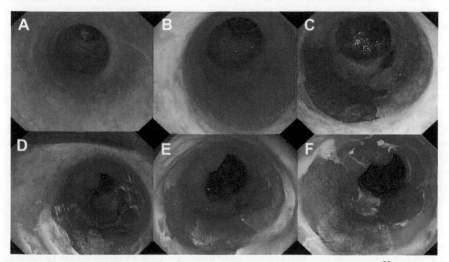

Fig. 5. Endoscopic appearance of a focal ablation procedure using the HALO^{90} system. (A) Antegrade view of an initial C6M7 Barrett esophagus 6 weeks after primary circumferential ablation. (B) Residual isles of Barrett mucosa. (C) Corresponding image with NBI. (D) Ablation effect immediately after ablation with the HALO^{90} system; the distal end of the catheter is visible at the 12 o'clock position in the endoscopic field. (E) Endoscopic appearance after the first ablation pass (2 × 15 J/cm^2) and cleaning of the ablation zones. (F) After the second ablation pass (2 × 15 J/cm^2), the ablation zones have a tan-colored appearance. (*Reproduced from* www.endosurgery.eu; with permission. *Courtesy of* ER and RFA Training Program, Amsterdam, The Netherlands; with permission.)

with suctioning away the debris through the working channel of the endoscope. This is followed by spraying off debris using the high-pressure pistol with plain water. Next, the endoscope with the HALO[90]-device is removed and coagulum is cleaned from the electrode using a wet gauze, taking care to wipe "with the grain" of the electrode array.

(5) Second ablation pass:

After cleaning, endoscope and HALO[90]-device are reintroduced and two more energy deliveries of 15 J/cm^2 are performed.

POSTPROCEDURAL CARE

Adequate acid-suppressant medication is key in the post-RFA treatment period to promote healing and re-epithelialization with normal squamous epithelium.[53–55] It is recommended to keep patients on a maintenance dosage of esomeprazole 40 mg twice a day during the entire treatment period. In our institution, patients are additionally prescribed ranitidine 300 mg at bedtime and sucralfate 1 g 4 times a day for a period of 14 days after each RFA treatment. Patients are advised to use a liquid diet during 24 hours after RFA, and to slowly return to normal diet normal thereafter. After RFA treatment, patients may experience chest pain and difficulty swallowing for 3 to 4 days. For pain management, viscous lidocaine, liquid acetaminophen with narcotic, or acetaminophen suppositories and antiemetics are used.

TREATMENT PROTOCOL AND FOLLOW-UP

RFA treatment is repeated every 2 to 3 months until all visible BE has been eradicated. Most studies have limited the number of RFA sessions to two HALO[360]- and three HALO[90]-procedures. Generally, patients will require one HALO[360]- and one or two HALO[90]-procedures. To assess whether all visible BE epithelium is removed, the use of high-resolution endoscopy with NBI (or comparable techniques such as iScan or Fujinon Intelligent Color Enhancement) is important, as this facilitates detection of small islands of residual BE epithelium that are easily overlooked with standard white light endoscopy.

Two months after the final treatment session, four quadrant biopsies are taken every 1 to 2 cm of the original BE segment to exclude the presence of buried Barrett's. Complete removal of BE can be difficult to assess endoscopically and when in doubt, biopsies should be taken immediately distal to the neosquamocolumnar junction to rule out residual intestinal metaplasia and/or dysplasia. After histology has confirmed the complete eradication of IM and dysplasia, patients are scheduled for follow-up endoscopy at 6 months, at 12 months, and annually thereafter.

In case of residual Barrett's islands after the maximum number of RFA sessions, further management can be subsequent HALO ablation, APC, or escape ER, left to the discretion of the endoscopist. When lesions suspicious for dysplasia or cancer are encountered during the RFA treatment period or at control endoscopy after RFA, directed biopsies should be obtained of the lesion with a low threshold to remove visible abnormalities by ER.

CHALLENGES IN RADIOFREQUENCY ABLATION

Although RFA with the HALO system is a simple and fast technique in most patients, occasionally more challenging RFA cases are encountered, eg, patients with a severely stenosed esophagus, a very long BE segment, or patients who show poor healing or poor regression of the BE epithelium. In patients with an esophageal stenosis (eg, a reflux stenosis at the upper end of the BE, or narrowing after widespread ER or prior ulceration in the BE) dilations should be performed to render patients eligible for RFA treatment. In case the EID varies over the length of the BE segment, treatment with two different HALO^{360}-balloon sizes is an option. For a focally narrowed esophagus, use of the HALO^{360}-balloon can be combined with the HALO^{90}-device in a single session in selected patients. Secondly, in patients with a very long BE segment it may be beneficial to treat the BE in two sessions to reduce patient discomfort and complication risk. A small subgroup of patients (<10% in our hands) may show delayed healing of the ablated area, requiring postponing the RFA session. Generally, these patients will also show a high rate of regeneration of BE instead of squamous mucosa. In these patients we confirm adherence to the prescribed medication, again exclude the use of any caustic comedication, and increase the dosage of antiacid medication (eg, esomeprazole 80 mg twice a day). Finally, there is a very small subset of patients in which RFA treatment fails because of poor regression of BE for unknown reasons.

RESULTS OF RADIOFREQUENCY ABLATION

Since the HALO system was introduced in 2003, several groups have evaluated the safety and efficacy of RFA for BE patients with and without dysplasia. The most important results will be discussed in the following sections.

DOSE-ESCALATION OF RADIOFREQUENCY ENERGY

After dose-escalation studies in the porcine model and in patients before esophagectomy,[56,57] the first large study to report the results of RFA for Barrett's esophagus was performed from 2003 to 2005 in patients with nondysplastic BE (Ablation of IM [AIM]-study). In this study, dose response and safety of the HALO^{360}-device was further tested. Because there were no dose-related adverse events, the dose-escalation phase (n = 32) was followed by an effectiveness phase (n = 70) using two applications of radiofrequency energy with an energy level of 10 J/cm^2. After 12 months of follow-up, complete eradication of IM was reached in 70% of 70 patients.[58]

FOCAL ABLATION COMES INTO PLAY

Once the HALO^{90}-device for focal ablation became available, much higher eradication rates for IM were reached. The HALO^{90}-device not only enables the precise targeting of small residual BE areas but also allows for effective treatment at the level of the gastroesophageal junction where the HALO^{360}-device may not always come in optimal contact with the epithelium.

The aforementioned AIM study incorporated HALO^{90} for focal ablation of residual BE in the study protocol and entered 62 patients in a study extension phase. Thirty months after the initial focal ablation, complete remission of IM was achieved in 98% of 61 available patients with a mean of two focal ablation procedures without serious adverse events or strictures. No buried Barrett's glands were detected in 4306 biopsies during the first 12 months and 923 biopsies collected at 30 months after primary circumferential ablation.[48]

INTRODUCTION IN EUROPE

After initial trials in the United States using a bottom-up approach, the promising RFA technique was also introduced in Europe. Our group was the first to use a combined treatment approach of ER followed by RFA for BE with early neoplasia (**Fig. 6**). In the

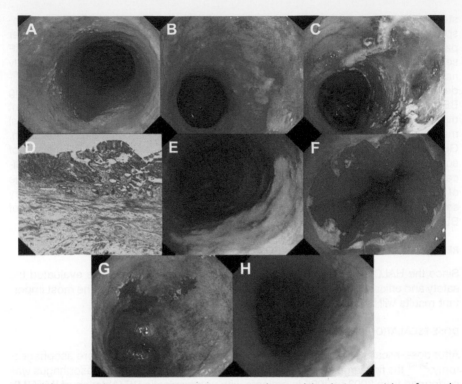

Fig. 6. (A) Antegrade view on a C6M10 Barrett esophagus. (B) A lesion suspicious for early cancer at the 2 to 4 o'clock position. (C) View on the resection wound after endoscopic resection of the lesion in two pieces. (D) Histopathological evaluation of the specimens showed a radically resected adenocarcinoma infiltrating in the muscularis mucosae (Hematoxylin and Eosin staining/40× magnification [T1m3]). (E) Same area 6 weeks after the endoscopic resection. The wound has healed completely with scarring. (F) Ablation effect after primary circumferential ablation using the HALO360 system (2 × 12 J/cm²). (G) Residual isle of Barrett mucosa remaining 6 weeks after prior circumferential ablation. (H) After additional focal ablation of residual isles of Barrett mucosa, complete removal of the whole Barrett segment was reached. (*Reproduced from* www.endosurgery.eu; with permission. *Courtesy of* ER and RFA Training Program, Amsterdam, The Netherlands; with permission.)

first series of 11 patients who underwent RFA for a median BE length of 5 cm, a prior "en bloc" ER was performed for visible lesions in 6 of 11 patients. The HALO⁹⁰-device was implemented in the second half of the study period and used at 12 and 15 J/cm². After a median follow-up of 14 months after initial ablation, 100% of the patients had been histologically cleared of all IM and dysplasia.[51] The second series of 12 patients also enrolled patients after a prior piecemeal resection of visible lesions. In this study, the ablation area and the electrode were cleaned between ablation passes.[50,52] Again, in 100% of patients, eradication of IM and dysplasia was reached, and although patients with a significantly longer BE were enrolled, fewer treatment sessions were required.

To study the functional characteristics of the normal-appearing esophagus after RFA, esophageal manometry and a functional lumen imaging probe (FLIP) were used, showing unchanged esophageal motility and compliance after RFA.[59]

RESULTS OF RADIOFREQUENCY ABLATION AFTER 2-YEAR FOLLOW-UP

Recently, our group reported the combined results of the first 44 patients with BE containing early neoplasia, treated with RFA with or without prior ER after a median follow-up of 21 months. In addition to the studies mentioned previously, patients from two other study protocols were included in this combined group: a series of 9 patients who participated in an ongoing European multicenter trial studying RFA for patients with BE less than 12 cm, and a series of 12 patients who were randomized to RFA in a study comparing radical endoscopic resection (RER) and RFA in patients with BE less than 5 cm. In these 44 patients of whom 31 underwent ER prior or RFA, the clearance rate of IM and dysplasia was 98% after a median follow-up of 21 months. No strictures were found.[31,51,52]

Sharma and colleagues[33] reported the single-center results of RFA for LGD (n = 39) and HGD (n = 24) with a median follow-up of 24 months. An overall clearance rate for dysplasia of 89%, and clearance rate for IM of 79% was achieved. In the HGD group, the clearance rate of HGD was 100%, whereas the clearance rate of all dysplasia was 79%, and the clearance rate for IM was 67%. In the LGD group, the clearance rate of all dysplasia was 95% and the clearance rate for IM was 87%. In this cohort, only 2 HGD patients underwent ER before RFA. There were no buried glands in 2500 biopsies.

MULTICENTER REGISTRATION

After the promising first results of treating HGD, a prospective multicenter registry was initiated in which 16 US centers participated. After 12 months of follow-up, complete eradication of HGD was achieved in 90% of 92 patients. The eradication rate of IM was only 54%, possibly because the HALO[90] was not yet used in this cohort. In this large series, only eight patients previously underwent ER. There were no serious adverse events, but there was one asymptomatic stenosis. Buried glands were not reported. The large number of patients and the multicenter set-up of this study show that RFA using the HALO[360]-device can be safely implemented in clinical practice.[60]

A RANDOMIZED CLINICAL TRIAL

Essential evidence that RFA is highly effective in the treatment of dysplastic Barrett's esophagus, comes from the multicenter AIM-Dysplasia trial.[61] In this trial, 127 patients with BE containing either LGD (n = 64) or HGD (n = 63) were randomized 2:1 to RFA or a sham procedure. Eleven patients underwent ER before RFA. Twelve months after the initial RFA treatment, patients underwent a biopsy session to assess if dysplasia and intestinal metaplasia were completely eradicated. In an intention to treat (ITT) analysis, 86% (92% per protocol [PP]) of RFA patients was cleared of dysplasia versus 21% (23% PP) of sham patients ($P<.001$). In the RFA arm, 77% (83% PP) of patients were completely cleared of IM versus 2% (3% PP) of sham patients ($P<.001$). In the HGD cohort separately, RFA patients showed a clearance rate of dysplasia of 81% (90% PP) versus 19% (20% PP) of sham patients ($P<.001$). The clearance rate of dysplasia in LGD patients was comparably high, with 90% (95% PP) of patients in the RFA arm cleared from dysplasia versus 23% (26% PP) in the sham arm ($P<.001$). For the HGD cohort, the progression rate was lower in the RFA arm, as in the RFA arm 1 of 42 patients developed carcinoma versus 4 of 21 patients in the sham arm ($P = .03$). This suggests that RFA changes the natural course of the disease.

The results of this important study confirm that RFA treatment of patients with HGD is safe and highly effective. Because of the randomized design, the study demonstrates that treatment with RFA for patients with HGD is more effective than 3-monthly surveillance endoscopies, making surveillance for patients with HGD no longer acceptable. The results also show that the use of other ablation techniques or surgery for patients with HGD in BE is questionable, as RFA is an excellent minimal-invasive alternative with a low complication rate.

ADVERSE EVENTS

RFA using the HALO system is associated with a low complication rate. After RFA treatment, patients have reported chest pain and difficulty swallowing for 3 to 4 days, which resolves spontaneously and can be adequately managed by pain medication. However, sporadically, patients with severe chest pain are admitted for observation and conservatively managed by optimizing pain medication and acid suppressants. Small nontransmural lacerations are sometimes observed during RFA procedures. We have recently analyzed all patients treated with RFA in our center, including patients who were treated with RFA out of study protocols. A nontransmural laceration was reported in 6% of the patients, and exclusively in patients with a prior ER and/or a balloon of a too-large diameter according to the rule of thumb "two sizes smaller than the smallest diameter in case of a prior ER." Also, some patients (8%) developed dysphagia resolving upon dilation, and this was encountered only in patients with an extended ER of more than 2 cm in size or comprising more than 50% of the circumference of the esophagus.[62] These findings underline the importance of limiting the extent of the ER, and it is likely that ongoing trials will provide more information on how to optimize the combination of ER and RFA. No perforations and no RFA-associated deaths were reported.[31,32,48,51,52,58,62] In summary, the complication profile of RFA compares favorably to that of other ablation techniques such as PDT and APC.[19,20,22]

CHARACTERISTICS OF THE NEOSQUAMOUS EPITHELIUM AFTER RADIOFREQUENCY ABLATION

One of the striking findings in all these clinical studies was the virtual absence of buried Barrett's glands (BBG) after RFA, whereas these are typically reported after all previously used ablation techniques in BE. Only in one RFA trial the presence of BBG after RFA was reported.[61] In the AIM-Dysplasia trial, comparing RFA versus a sham procedure in patients with dysplastic BE, 25.2% of patients had BBG at baseline, which was reduced to 5.1% at 12 months after RFA, whereas in the sham arm there was an increase in the rate of BBG, that were present in 40% of patients. The use of an aggressive biopsy protocol only during follow-up (four quadrant jumbo biopsies each 1 cm) could address this rise in the rate of BBG in patients in the sham arm. It has been suggested that in other studies BBG were not detected, because of less deep biopsy sampling in the theoretically altered mucosa after RFA. Our group conducted a study to assess biopsy depth and presence of BBG after RFA. Biopsies and ER specimens were obtained from neosquamous and untreated squamous epithelium from patients treated with RFA for BE containing early neoplasia.[63] Blind assessment by three expert pathologists showed no difference in biopsy depth between the neosquamous and untreated squamous epithelium and in none of the biopsies or ER specimens were BBG found. This study also evaluated the presence of oncogenetic abnormalities in the BE epithelium before and after RFA. Fluorescent in situ hybridization (FISH) of brush cytology specimens and immunohistological evaluation of biopsies obtained from the BE epithelium at baseline and from the neosquamous epithelium after RFA showed absence of preexisting oncogenetic alterations, which was confirmed by others.[64] The absence of BBG and oncogenetic alterations in the newly formed squamous epithelial lining suggests that the risk for malignant progression in these patients is reduced to the normal level of individuals without BE.

RADIOFREQUENCY ABLATION FOR LOW-GRADE DYSPLASIA

Some of the previously mentioned clinical trials have also enrolled patients with LGD in Barrett's esophagus, although current guidelines advise endoscopic surveillance with an interval of 6 to 12 months.[34,65] RFA for LGD is controversial, as the risk for malignant progression is considered to be smaller than in HGD.[34] There is a large spread in reported progression rates to cancer for LGD in BE, varying from 1% to 46%.[66–69] The main reason for this is the poor interobserver agreement for the diagnosis LGD: inflammatory reactive changes are easily misinterpreted as dysplasia. In case a patient is diagnosed with LGD, it is therefore advised to have histology reviewed by an expert pathologist, to risk-stratify patients correctly. Many patients with presumed LGD are down-graded to nondysplastic BE by the expert pathologist, whereas a consensus diagnosis of LGD between two or more expert pathologists is associated with a high risk for progression, varying from 16% to 28%.[67,70,71] In our opinion, the impressive efficacy and safety profile of RFA justify its use in patients with a consensus diagnosis of LGD.

ISSUES AND FUTURE PROSPECTS

Endoscopic treatment is currently the therapy of choice in the Western world for selected patients with HGD or mucosal cancer in BE. The combination of ER of visible abnormalities and RFA is clearly superior to other available treatment modalities. The reported success rates for eradication of HGD vary between 81% and 100% and complete removal of IM is reported in 67% to 100% of cases, without recurrences of IM or dysplasia during follow-up.[31,32,48,51,52,61] More results of several European and American clinical trials are currently under way. There are several issues that can be objectives for further research.

The first and most important issue is the lack of long-term results on the outcome of patients after RFA treatment. Longest reported follow-up periods are 21 months for cohort of Barrett's patients with HGD or cancer,[31] 24 months for a cohort of Barrett's patients with LGD or HGD,[32] and 30 months for nondysplastic Barrett's patients.[48]

Another main issue is whether or not RFA is indicated in nondysplastic BE. This is will be dependent on the durability of eradication of Barrett's epithelium. When complete remission of IM and dysplasia are found to be permanent, cost-effectiveness studies suggest that RFA is the dominant strategy over surveillance.[72] Ongoing basic research focusing on prognostic biomarkers may contribute in the identification of nondysplastic BE patients with an increased risk for progressing to HGD or cancer in whom RFA would then be a logical preventive measure.

An aspect that needs to be addressed is the relevance of IM present below the neo-Z-line. Currently in all patients the Z-line is treated circumferentially using the HALO90-device in the subsequent RFA session to treat endoscopically invisible BE. Despite this approach, intestinal metaplasia has been detected in biopsies taken immediately below the neo-Z-line in the gastric cardia in few patients.[31] The clinical relevance of IM distal to the neo-Z-line is unclear. Some may argue that this reflects residual Barrett's, whereas others refer to the presence of nondysplastic IM of the cardia in 25% of individuals without BE and the fact that a malignant potential for nondysplastic IM in the cardia has not been shown.[73] In our opinion, IM of the cardia that is found during follow-up after RFA is not an indication for repeated treatment.

An interesting question is where the neosquamous epithelium after RFA has its origin. Although in the neosquamous epithelium the preexisting oncogenetic abnormalities of BE epithelium were absent,[63,64] more knowledge on the nature and source of neosquamous cells may unravel if the neosquamous lining truly holds a low risk for malignant progression. It has been suggested that repopulation is established by migration of squamous stem cells from adjacent squamous epithelium, or by differentiation of regional squamous progenitors or circulating stem cells.[54,74,75] New knowledge on the process of re-epithelialization may also explain why sporadically patients fail to respond to RFA treatment. Also, identification of factors that predict a poor response to RFA may be helpful to optimize success rates of RFA treatment.

Last, it is questionable if every endoscopist should be trained in RFA. Although this novel ablation technique is relatively easy to apply, RFA is just one aspect in the whole spectrum of endoscopic management of BE patients. Selection of patients with a proper indication for RFA involves thorough endoscopic work-up, the possibility to safely perform ER, and accurate histologic evaluation of tissue specimens for the presence of risk factors for lymph node metastasis. We think that RFA should, therefore, be centralized in centers with multidisciplinary expertise in this field. To realize this, adequate training courses (eg, www.endosurgery.eu), aimed at the whole spectrum of endoscopic management, are mandatory to maintain the status of endoscopic treatment as a valid and safe alternative to surgical treatment in the management of early Barrett neoplasia.

SUMMARY

RFA is a novel and promising treatment modality in the treatment of BE with HGD or mucosal cancer, and is not associated with stenosis or buried glandular mucosa, which are known side effects from other ablation techniques such as PDT and APC. The combination of ER followed by RFA for removal of the residual flat BE is a powerful management strategy. Several clinical trials have shown that RFA is safe and highly effective for the removal of dysplasia and complete conversion of the BE into normal-appearing squamous esophagus. Although no long-term results are available yet, RFA should be regarded as the treatment of choice in patients with early neoplasia in BE with or without a prior ER. Future research will focus on the natural course of dysplastic and nondysplastic BE, biomarkers predicting disease progression, and cost-effectiveness plus quality of life to assess if RFA treatment is justified for patients with nondysplastic BE.

REFERENCES

1. Spechler SJ. Clinical practice. Barrett's esophagus. N Engl J Med 2002;346(11): 836–42.
2. Sharma P, Sidorenko EI. Are screening and surveillance for Barrett's oesophagus really worthwhile? Gut 2005;54(Suppl 1):i27–32.
3. Haggitt RC, Tryzelaar J, Ellis FH, et al. Adenocarcinoma complicating columnar epithelium-lined (Barrett's) esophagus. Am J Clin Pathol 1978;70(1):1–5.
4. Haggitt RC. Barrett's esophagus, dysplasia, and adenocarcinoma. Hum Pathol 1994;25(10):982–93.
5. Haggitt RC. Pathology of Barrett's esophagus. J Gastrointest Surg 2000;4(2): 117–8.
6. Drewitz DJ, Sampliner RE, Garewal HS. The incidence of adenocarcinoma in Barrett's esophagus: a prospective study of 170 patients followed 4.8 years. Am J Gastroenterol 1997;92(2):212–5.

7. Hameeteman W, Tytgat GN, Houthoff HJ, et al. Barrett's esophagus: development of dysplasia and adenocarcinoma. Gastroenterology 1989;96(5 Pt 1):1249–56.

8. Shaheen NJ, Crosby MA, Bozymski EM, et al. Is there publication bias in the reporting of cancer risk in Barrett's esophagus? Gastroenterology 2000;119(2):333–8.

9. Chan WH, Wong WK, Chan HS, et al. Results of surgical resection of oesophageal carcinoma in Singapore. Ann Acad Med Singapore 2000;29(1):57–61.

10. Gillison EW, Powell J, McConkey CC, et al. Surgical workload and outcome after resection for carcinoma of the oesophagus and cardia. Br J Surg 2002;89(3):344–8.

11. Liu JF, Wang QZ, Hou J. Surgical treatment for cancer of the oesophagus and gastric cardia in Hebei, China. Br J Surg 2004;91(1):90–8.

12. Holscher AH, Bollschweiler E, Schneider PM, et al. Early adenocarcinoma in Barrett's oesophagus. Br J Surg 1997;84(10):1470–3.

13. Rice TW, Falk GW, Achkar E, et al. Surgical management of high-grade dysplasia in Barrett's esophagus. Am J Gastroenterol 1993;88(11):1832–6.

14. Thomas P, Doddoli C, Neville P, et al. Esophageal cancer resection in the elderly. Eur J Cardiothorac Surg 1996;10(11):941–6.

15. Buskens CJ, Westerterp M, Lagarde SM, et al. Prediction of appropriateness of local endoscopic treatment for high-grade dysplasia and early adenocarcinoma by EUS and histopathologic features. Gastrointest Endosc 2004;60(5):703–10.

16. Westerterp M, Koppert LB, Buskens CJ, et al. Outcome of surgical treatment for early adenocarcinoma of the esophagus or gastro-esophageal junction. Virchows Arch 2005;446(5):497–504.

17. Ell C, May A, Pech O, et al. Curative endoscopic resection of early esophageal adenocarcinomas (Barrett's cancer). Gastrointest Endosc 2007;65(1):3–10.

18. May A, Gossner L, Pech O, et al. Local endoscopic therapy for intraepithelial high-grade neoplasia and early adenocarcinoma in Barrett's oesophagus: acute-phase and intermediate results of a new treatment approach. Eur J Gastroenterol Hepatol 2002;14(10):1085–91.

19. Overholt BF, Panjehpour M, Halberg DL. Photodynamic therapy for Barrett's esophagus with dysplasia and/or early stage carcinoma: long-term results. Gastrointest Endosc 2003;58(2):183–8.

20. Peters F, Kara M, Rosmolen W, et al. Poor results of 5-aminolevulinic acid-photodynamic therapy for residual high-grade dysplasia and early cancer in Barrett esophagus after endoscopic resection. Endoscopy 2005;37(5):418–24.

21. Hage M, Siersema PD, Vissers KJ, et al. Genomic analysis of Barrett's esophagus after ablative therapy: persistence of genetic alterations at tumor suppressor loci. Int J Cancer 2006;118(1):155–60.

22. Krishnadath KK, Wang KK, Taniguchi K, et al. Persistent genetic abnormalities in Barrett's esophagus after photodynamic therapy. Gastroenterology 2000;119(3):624–30.

23. Hornick JL, Blount PL, Sanchez CA, et al. Biologic properties of columnar epithelium underneath reepithelialized squamous mucosa in Barrett's esophagus. Am J Surg Pathol 2005;29(3):372–80.

24. Van Laethem JL, Peny MO, Salmon I, et al. Intramucosal adenocarcinoma arising under squamous re-epithelialisation of Barrett's oesophagus. Gut 2000;46(4):574–7.

25. Overholt BF, Lightdale CJ, Wang KK, et al. Photodynamic therapy with porfimer sodium for ablation of high-grade dysplasia in Barrett's esophagus: international,

partially blinded, randomized phase III trial. Gastrointest Endosc 2005;62(4): 488–98.

26. Larghi A, Lightdale CJ, Ross AS, et al. Long-term follow-up of complete Barrett's eradication endoscopic mucosal resection (CBE-EMR) for the treatment of high grade dysplasia and intramucosal carcinoma. Endoscopy 2007; 39(12):1086–91.

27. Peters FP, Kara MA, Rosmolen WD, et al. Stepwise radical endoscopic resection is effective for complete removal of Barrett's esophagus with early neoplasia: a prospective study. Am J Gastroenterol 2006;101(7):1449–57.

28. Peters FP, Krishnadath KK, Rygiel AM, et al. Stepwise radical endoscopic resection of the complete Barrett's esophagus with early neoplasia successfully eradicates pre-existing genetic abnormalities. Am J Gastroenterol 2007;102(9):1853–61.

29. Pouw RE, Peters FP, Sempoux C, et al. Stepwise radical endoscopic resection for Barrett's esophagus with early neoplasia: report on a Brussels' cohort. Endoscopy 2008;40(11):892–8.

30. Seewald S, Akaraviputh T, Seitz U, et al. Circumferential EMR and complete removal of Barrett's epithelium: a new approach to management of Barrett's esophagus containing high-grade intraepithelial neoplasia and intramucosal carcinoma. Gastrointest Endosc 2003;57(7):854–9.

31. Pouw RE, Gondrie JJ, Sondermeijer CM, et al. Eradication of Barrett esophagus with early neoplasia by radiofrequency ablation, with or without endoscopic resection. J Gastrointest Surg 2008;12(10):1627–36.

32. Sharma VK, Jae KH, Das A, et al. Circumferential and focal ablation of Barrett's esophagus containing dysplasia. Am J Gastroenterol 2009;104(2):310–7.

33. Bollschweiler E, Baldus SE, Schroder W, et al. High rate of lymph-node metastasis in submucosal esophageal squamous-cell carcinomas and adenocarcinomas. Endoscopy 2006;38(2):149–56.

34. Sampliner RE. Updated guidelines for the diagnosis, surveillance, and therapy of Barrett's esophagus. Am J Gastroenterol 2002;97(8):1888–95.

35. The Paris endoscopic classification of superficial neoplastic lesions: esophagus, stomach, and colon: November 30 to December 1, 2002. Gastrointest Endosc 2003;58(Suppl 6):S3–43.

36. Update on the Paris classification of superficial neoplastic lesions in the digestive tract. Endoscopy 2005;37(6):570–8.

37. Sharma P, Dent J, Armstrong D, et al. The development and validation of an endoscopic grading system for Barrett's esophagus: the Prague C & M criteria. Gastroenterology 2006;131(5):1392–9.

38. Reid BJ, Blount PL, Feng Z, et al. Optimizing endoscopic biopsy detection of early cancers in Barrett's high-grade dysplasia. Am J Gastroenterol 2000; 95(11):3089–96.

39. Bergman JJ, Fockens P. Endoscopic ultrasonography in patients with gastroesophageal cancer. Eur J Ultrasound 1999;10(2–3):127–38.

40. Kelly S, Harris KM, Berry E, et al. A systematic review of the staging performance of endoscopic ultrasound in gastro-oesophageal carcinoma. Gut 2001;49(4): 534–9.

41. Pech O, May A, Gunter E, et al. The impact of endoscopic ultrasound and computed tomography on the TNM staging of early cancer in Barrett's esophagus. Am J Gastroenterol 2006;101(10):2223–9.

42. May A, Gunter E, Roth F, et al. Accuracy of staging in early oesophageal cancer using high resolution endoscopy and high resolution endosonography: a comparative, prospective, and blinded trial. Gut 2004;53(5):634–40.

43. Muthusamy R, Rastogi A, Edmundowicz S, et al. The utility of Endoscopic Ultrasound (EUS) in patients with Barrett's esophagus (BE) and high grade dysplasia (HGD): analysis of the AIM Dysplasia trial experience [abstract]. Gastrointest Endosc 2008;67(5):AB99.
44. Peters FP, Kara MA, Curvers WL, et al. Multiband mucosectomy for endoscopic resection of Barrett's esophagus: feasibility study with matched historical controls. Eur J Gastroenterol Hepatol 2007;19(4):311–5.
45. Peters FP, Brakenhoff KP, Curvers WL, et al. Endoscopic cap resection for treatment of early Barrett's neoplasia is safe: a prospective analysis of acute and early complications in 216 procedures. Dis Esophagus 2007;20(6):510–5.
46. Schlemper RJ, Riddell RH, Kato Y, et al. The Vienna classification of gastrointestinal epithelial neoplasia. Gut 2000;47(2):251–5.
47. Schlemper RJ, Kato Y, Stolte M. Diagnostic criteria for gastrointestinal carcinomas in Japan and Western countries: proposal for a new classification system of gastrointestinal epithelial neoplasia. J Gastroenterol Hepatol 2000; (Suppl 15):G49–57.
48. Fleischer DE, Overholt BF, Sharma VK, et al. Endoscopic ablation of Barrett's esophagus: a multicenter study with 2.5-year follow-up. Gastrointest Endosc 2008;68(5):867–76.
49. Sharma VK, Kim HJ, Das A, et al. A prospective pilot trial of ablation of Barrett's esophagus with low-grade dysplasia using stepwise circumferential and focal ablation (HALO system). Endoscopy 2008;40(5):380–7.
50. Gondrie JJ, Pouw RE, Sondermeijer CM, et al. Optimizing the technique for circumferential ablation of Barrett esophagus containing high-grade dysplasia using the HALO360 System [abstract]. Gastrointest Endosc 2007;65(5):AB151.
51. Gondrie JJ, Pouw RE, Sondermeijer CM, et al. Stepwise circumferential and focal ablation of Barrett's esophagus with high-grade dysplasia: results of the first prospective series of 11 patients. Endoscopy 2008;40(5):359–69.
52. Gondrie JJ, Pouw RE, Sondermeijer CM, et al. Effective treatment of early Barrett's neoplasia with stepwise circumferential and focal ablation using the HALO system. Endoscopy 2008;40(5):370–9.
53. Barham CP, Jones RL, Biddlestone LR, et al. Photothermal laser ablation of Barrett's oesophagus: endoscopic and histological evidence of squamous re-epithelialisation. Gut 1997;41(3):281–4.
54. Berenson MM, Johnson TD, Markowitz NR, et al. Restoration of squamous mucosa after ablation of Barrett's esophageal epithelium. Gastroenterology 1993;104(6):1686–91.
55. Sampliner RE, Hixson LJ, Fennerty MB, et al. Regression of Barrett's esophagus by laser ablation in an acid environment. Dig Dis Sci 1993;38(2):365–8.
56. Dunkin BJ, Martinez J, Bejarano PA, et al. Thin-layer ablation of human esophageal epithelium using a bipolar radiofrequency balloon device. Surg Endosc 2006;20(1):125–30.
57. Ganz RA, Utley DS, Stern RA, et al. Complete ablation of esophageal epithelium with a balloon-based bipolar electrode: a phased evaluation in the porcine and in the human esophagus. Gastrointest Endosc 2004;60(6):1002–10.
58. Sharma VK, Wang KK, Overholt BF, et al. Balloon-based, circumferential, endoscopic radiofrequency ablation of Barrett's esophagus: 1-year follow-up of 100 patients. Gastrointest Endosc 2007;65(2):185–95.
59. Beaumont H, Gondrie JJ, McMahon BP, et al. Stepwise radiofrequency ablation of Barrett's esophagus preserves esophageal inner diameter, compliance, and motility. Endoscopy 2009;41(1):2–8.

60. Ganz RA, Overholt BF, Sharma VK, et al. Circumferential ablation of Barrett's esophagus that contains high-grade dysplasia: a U.S. Multicenter Registry. Gastrointest Endosc 2008;68(1):35–40.
61. Shaheen NJ, Sharma P, Overholt BF, et al. Radiofrequency ablation in Barrett's esophagus with dysplasia. N Engl J Med 2009;360(22):2277–88.
62. Pouw RE, Gondrie JJ, van Vilsteren FGI, et al. Complications following circumferential Radiofrequency energy ablation of Barrett's esophagus containing early neoplasia [abstract]. Gastrointest Endosc 2008;67(5):AB145.
63. Pouw RE, Gondrie JJ, Rygiel AM, et al. Properties of the neosquamous epithelium after radiofrequency ablation of Barrett's esophagus containing neoplasia. Am J Gastroenterol 2009;104(6):1366–73.
64. Finkelstein SD, Lyday WD. The molecular pathology of radiofrequency mucosal ablation of Barrett's esophagus [abstract]. Gastroenterology 2008;134(Suppl 4): A436.
65. Hirota WK, Zuckerman MJ, Adler DG, et al. ASGE guideline: the role of endoscopy in the surveillance of premalignant conditions of the upper GI tract. Gastrointest Endosc 2006;63(4):570–80.
66. Schnell TG, Sontag SJ, Chejfec G, et al. Long-term nonsurgical management of Barrett's esophagus with high-grade dysplasia. Gastroenterology 2001;120(7): 1607–19.
67. Montgomery E, Bronner MP, Goldblum JR, et al. Reproducibility of the diagnosis of dysplasia in Barrett esophagus: a reaffirmation. Hum Pathol 2001;32(4): 368–78.
68. Reid BJ, Levine DS, Longton G, et al. Predictors of progression to cancer in Barrett's esophagus: baseline histology and flow cytometry identify low- and high-risk patient subsets. Am J Gastroenterol 2000;95(7):1669–76.
69. Wani S, Mathur S, Sharma P. How to manage a Barrett's esophagus patient with low-grade dysplasia. Clin Gastroenterol Hepatol 2009;7(1):27–32.
70. Curvers WL, Rosmolen WD, Elzer B, et al. Low-grade intra-epithelial in Barrett's esophagus: over-diagnosed but underestimated [abstract]. Gastrointest Endosc 2008;67(5):AB181.
71. Skacel M, Petras RE, Gramlich TL, et al. The diagnosis of low-grade dysplasia in Barrett's esophagus and its implications for disease progression. Am J Gastroenterol 2000;95(12):3383–7.
72. Inadomi JM, Somsouk M, Madanick RD, et al. A cost-utility analysis of ablative therapy for Barrett's esophagus. Gastroenterology 2009;136(7):2101–14.
73. Morales TG, Camargo E, Bhattacharyya A, et al. Long-term follow-up of intestinal metaplasia of the gastric cardia. Am J Gastroenterol 2000;95(7):1677–80.
74. Paulson TG, Xu L, Sanchez C, et al. Neosquamous epithelium does not typically arise from Barrett's epithelium. Clin Cancer Res 2006;12(6):1701–6.
75. Sarosi G, Brown G, Jaiswal K, et al. Bone marrow progenitor cells contribute to esophageal regeneration and metaplasia in a rat model of Barrett's esophagus. Dis Esophagus 2008;21(1):43–50.

Cryotherapy in the Management of Esophageal Dysplasia and Malignancy

Kevin D. Halsey, MD, Bruce D. Greenwald, MD*

KEYWORDS

- Esophageal adenocarcinoma • Barrett metaplasia
- High-grade dysplasia • Cryotherapy • Endoscopic therapy

Barrett esophagus is a premalignant condition in which normal stratified squamous epithelium of the esophagus is replaced by metaplastic columnar epithelium.[1] Chronic esophageal reflux is believed to be responsible for this mucosal transformation.[2,3] Dysplasia arising within metaplastic epithelium is recognized as the major risk factor leading to the development of adenocarcinoma. Dysplasia is believed to progress from low-grade dysplasia to high-grade dysplasia (HGD), and ultimately transform into esophageal adenocarcinoma.[4,5] Esophageal cancer remains relatively uncommon, yet its incidence has continued to rise steadily over the last 3 decades.[6,7] In 2008, approximately 16,000 patients (12,500 men and 3500 women) were diagnosed with esophageal cancer and nearly 14,000 died from the disease.[8] These patients generally have a poor prognosis with an overall 5-year survival rate of 10% to 15%.[9]

Healthy patients with biopsy-proven HGD typically have been treated with esophagectomy because of a 5% to 6% annual risk of developing esophageal adenocarcinoma.[10] Many patients are determined to be poor surgical candidates, making it difficult to justify the morbidity and mortality associated with esophagectomy.[11] This has led to the development of several methods of controlled mucosal ablation with the goal of preventing the development of esophageal adenocarcinoma. Currently, endoscopic ablation of Barrett esophagus with HGD and intramucosal carcinoma (IMCA) is accepted therapy for those patients considered inoperable or who decline

Financial disclosures: Dr Greenwald is a consultant and receives research funding from CSA Medical, Inc. Dr Halsey has nothing to disclose.
Division of Gastroenterology and Hepatology, Department of Medicine, University of Maryland School of Medicine, 22 South Greene Street, N3W62, MD 21201-1595, USA
* Corresponding author.
E-mail address: bgreenwa@medicine.umaryland.edu (B.D. Greenwald).

surgical therapy, and studies have shown that elimination of HGD significantly lessens the risk of developing esophageal adenocarcinoma.[12]

Current ablative techniques include endoscopic resection,[13] photodynamic therapy (PDT),[14,15] argon plasma coagulation (APC),[16,17] Nd:YAG (neodymium:yttrium-aluminum-garnet) laser,[18] multipolar electrocoagulation,[19] balloon- and catheter-based radiofrequency ablation (RFA),[20,21] and cryotherapy. These techniques have achieved mucosal ablation with variable success and each has unique advantages and disadvantages. This article highlights the cumulative findings on the efficacy and safety of cryotherapy in the treatment of esophageal dysplasia and carcinoma.

MECHANISM OF ACTION

Cryotherapy is the application of extreme cold to biologic tissues for medical treatment. Studies have shown it is most effective when administered as repeated cycles of rapid freezing followed by slow thawing.[22,23] This process destroys tissue through a combination of immediate and delayed effects while also preserving the cryoresistant structures of the extracellular matrix.[24] Initial cooling causes hypothermia, which stresses cell proteins and lipids. Ultimately, this can lead to cell death even if freezing temperatures are not reached. When tissue temperatures reach freezing, extracellular water freezes, forming ice crystals. These extracellular ice crystals create a hyperosmotic environment, drawing water from intracellular compartments. As the temperature continues to fall, crystallization accelerates, amplifying fluid shifts and resulting in cellular shrinkage and destruction of cellular membranes and organelles (solution-effect injury). Rapid freezing and lower temperatures favor formation of intracellular ice, increasing the likelihood of cell death. Colder temperatures appear to be needed to reliably destroy cancer cells and increase the likelihood of destroying all cells in the treated area.

During the thawing portion of the treatment cycle, large crystals form and disrupt cellular membranes through mechanical and shearing forces. Further membrane disruption occurs as ice crystals melt, producing a hypotonic extracellular environment that shifts water back into cells and ruptures cell membranes. Tissue hypothermia remains for minutes following complete thawing, subjecting tissues to continued metabolic injury.

Vascular stasis, with tissue ischemia and anoxia, is instrumental in cryotherapy-induced tissue destruction. Initial cooling results in vasoconstriction and decreased blood flow, and freezing produces cessation of blood flow. Thawing produces vasodilation and increased vascular permeability through endothelial damage. This damage results in edema, platelet aggregation, and formation of microthrombi, leading to further circulatory collapse. Continued microcirculatory occlusion results in uniform cell death in the affected area, including cells that may have survived the initial insult.

Repetition of the freeze-thaw cycle results in greater cellular destruction. Tissue cooling is more rapid with each cycle, and the volume of frozen tissue is increased as the cryoeffect further penetrates the target tissue. This results in greater extent, depth, and volume of destroyed tissue in a dose-dependent manner. Relative resistance of stromal components to freezing injury (including collagen fibers) leads to favorable healing[24] because preservation of the extracellular matrix results in a more controlled wound response with less potential for fibrosis and scarring.[25]

Induction of an immunologic reaction is one of the most intriguing aspects of cryotherapy. This technique has been shown to induce cellular apoptosis in cancer cells and may lead to death of malignant cells outside of the original treatment area.[26,27]

This characteristic, unique to cryotherapy, makes cryotherapy particularly useful and attractive in the treatment of Barrett-associated HGD and cancer, as inhibition of apoptosis is one element involved in pathogenesis.[28,29] Apoptosis-induced immunogenicity can lead hypothetically to an established cellular immunity within esophageal mucosa capable of killing malignant cells that develop long after cryotherapy has been completed.[30]

CRYOTHERAPY SYSTEMS

Different agents, known as cryogens, have undergone clinical investigation to assess their success at tissue destruction. Liquid nitrogen is inert, inexpensive, and readily available, and it has been used successfully as a cryogen for over 5 decades, given its reliability and known effects.[31] It can cool tissues to approximately $-196°C$. Carbon dioxide (CO_2) is another cryogen used for gastrointestinal indications. CO_2-based cryotherapy uses the rapid high-pressure expansion of CO_2 to induce rapid cooling of tissues to approximately $-78°C$ (the Joule-Thompson effect).[32]

Two separate noncontact catheter-based systems have been developed for spraying cryogen through the working channel of an endoscope. In both, the operator uses the duration of cryogen application and time of tissue freezing to control the depth of esophageal injury. The Cryospray Ablation System (CSA Medical, Inc, Baltimore, Maryland) is a low–ambient pressure system using liquid nitrogen (**Fig. 1**). A 7F

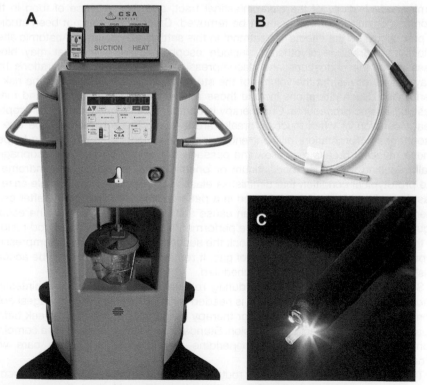

Fig. 1. Equipment used for endoscopic spray cryotherapy with liquid nitrogen. (*A*) Integrated console. (*B*) Cryo-decompression tube. (*C*) A 7F catheter in the channel of a diagnostic endoscope. (*Courtesy of* CSA Medical, Inc, Baltimore, MD; with permission.)

catheter is passed through the working channel of a standard upper endoscope, and the pressure exiting the distal tip of the catheter is approximately 2 to 4 psi. The console consists of a holding tank for liquid nitrogen and the electronic controls necessary to control flow of the cryogen. The console contains a timer with visual and auditory cues to monitor spray time and counters to track the number of freeze-thaw cycles and sites treated. A heating circuit warms the catheter at the end of the procedure to ease removal from the scope. External suction from a pump or wall suction is controlled within the console and connected to an orogastric decompression tube (described below). A two-pedal foot switch is provided with the system—one to activate the spray and the other to engage and disengage suction. Treatment is performed under direct endoscopic visualization and the extent of therapy is controlled by the operator using the foot pedal to control duration of spray.

The Polar Wand cryotherapy device (GI Supply, Camp Hill, Pennsylvania) is a delivery system using CO_2 to generate a cryogen. Rapidly expanding high-pressure CO_2 gas produces cooling, known as the Joule-Thompson effect. A catheter is passed through the working channel of an upper endoscope, and a suction catheter is attached to the tip of the endoscope for decompression throughout the procedure.

TREATMENT TECHNIQUE

There are several contraindications to spray cryotherapy, including pregnancy, anatomic alterations of the esophagus or stomach, breaks in the esophageal mucosa, diminished elasticity of the gastrointestinal tract, and the presence of food in the stomach or duodenum that cannot be removed. Cryotherapy has not been studied in pregnancy, so the effects of treatment in this setting are unknown. Anatomic alterations that preclude cryotherapy include esophageal narrowing that may block passage of the endoscope and decompression tube and gastric alterations that may reduce or restrict the volume of the stomach, potentially increasing the risk of perforation. Such alterations include those related to gastrojejunostomy and many gastric bariatric procedures. Cryotherapy is contraindicated in the setting of esophageal ulceration or when mucosal breaks are evident. These breaks can be due to esophageal inflammation, dilation, endoscopic resection, or an aggressive biopsy. These mucosal breaks may allow the passage of cryogen through the esophageal wall, resulting in pneumomediastinum or pneumoperitoneum. Marfan syndrome is the prototypical condition that diminishes elasticity of the stomach. A single case of gastric perforation has been reported in a patient with Marfan syndrome after cryotherapy. Eosinophilic esophagitis can cause stiffening and narrowing of the esophagus, and cryotherapy should not be performed in advanced disease. Food residue in the stomach or duodenum may block the suction ports in the cryo-decompression tube and prevent adequate venting of gas. If removal of this food cannot be accomplished, the procedure must be rescheduled.

Spray cryotherapy is performed during routine outpatient upper gastrointestinal endoscopy. No specific preparation is needed for cryotherapy. For esophageal ablation, high-dose proton pump inhibitor therapy (twice daily) is initiated 1 week before treatment to maximize acid suppression. Standard sedation is used, either a combination of midazolam and fentanyl/meperidine or monitored anesthesia care with propofol.

Treatment sessions begin with routine endoscopic evaluation. Before scope removal, a guidewire (typically a Savary-Gilliard wire [Cook Medical, Bloomington, Indiana]) is inserted through the scope and left with the distal tip in the stomach. After scope removal, the cryo-decompression tube is lubricated and inserted over the wire into the stomach. Liquid nitrogen spray generates 6 to 8 L of nitrogen gas during a 20-second treatment as the expelled liquid expands into a gas. This tube allows rapid gastric decompression and removal of sprayed nitrogen during treatment cycles. The tube itself contains multiple side holes for luminal decompression. Active suction occurs in the distal tube, demarcated by a double black line on the tube itself. Side holes in the proximal tube open in the esophagus and passively vent to the air for esophageal decompression. Before scope reinsertion, a soft clear friction-fit cap (eg, D-201-11804 [Olympus America, Center Valley, Pennsylvania]) is inserted over the tip of the endoscope to optimize visualization and prevent the cryocatheter tip from contacting the mucosa. The endoscope is reinserted and advanced to the distal esophagus. The decompression tube is withdrawn until the black line on the tube approximates the gastroesophageal junction. The scope is then positioned to the treatment area and the cryocatheter is passed through the biopsy channel and advanced just distal to the tip of the endoscope, allowing for enough clearance to avoid frosting of the lens on the end of the endoscope.

Suction is activated before each cryogen application via the foot pedal. Targeted tissue is frozen for the appropriate length of time (typically 10–20 seconds) and allowed to thaw, thus completing one cycle of treatment. Typically, a targeted area is treated for two to four cycles. If the entire area of interest has not been treated, the next site is selected and the freeze-thaw cycles are repeated. While spraying, the patient is monitored by endoscopy personnel for abdominal distension by placing a hand on the patient's abdomen. The procedure is temporarily halted if abdominal distension is noted or if suction is compromised.

The surface area of the esophagus that can be kept frozen during a treatment cycle is variable and is determined by the physician. An area 3 cm across can easily be kept frozen for the needed time. Hemicircumferential or circumferential freezing is also possible, especially in later treatment cycles and sites, where the area is already hypothermic (**Fig. 2**). Overlap areas between two treatment sites occur routinely. Once treatment is complete, the scope and cryo-decompression tube are removed from the patient. Removal of the catheter from the scope is aided by using the heat cycle provided on the console to warm the catheter and scope. Cryotherapy has been

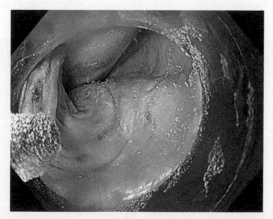

Fig. 2. Endoscopic appearance of tissue freezing during spray cryotherapy in the esophagus. The spray catheter is seen on the left side of the image and the cryo-decompression tube is visible at the top of the picture. A clear friction-fit cap is fitted over the tip of the endoscope.

used extensively at some centers since 2006, and no damage to endoscopes has been reported despite multiple uses.

Treatment sessions typically are repeated every 6 to 8 weeks until the area of interest has completely regressed (**Figs. 3** and **4**). Incomplete healing may be seen if the treatment interval is too short, and twice-daily proton pump inhibitor is continued until all treatment is complete. Patients are given prescriptions for pain and medications for nausea, but they typically are not needed. A topical anesthetic mixture ("magic mouthwash") containing lidocaine solution is prescribed for painful swallowing and is helpful to some patients.

Inherent difficulties at targeting areas of interest include fogging of the scope lens, maneuvering the cryocatheter to treat areas covered by the decompression tube, and maintaining adequate abdominal decompression. In the majority of cases, these difficulties do not prevent complete treatment. A common error made by new users is to begin timing the tissue freeze as soon as any frost is seen on the tissue. This leads to undertreatment and inadequate results. The freeze timer should not be started until the entire targeted area is covered by the ice field. Another potential error is to begin a new cycle of freezing before the tissue has completely thawed. As discussed above, the thaw portion of the treatment cycle is as important as freezing, and the tissue must be allowed to thaw completely before being refrozen.

DOSIMETRY

Dosimetry is controlled by freeze time and number of freeze-thaw cycles performed. Animal studies using the swine model have been conducted both for the liquid nitrogen and CO_2 systems. In a comparison between APC, multipolar electrocoagulation, and liquid nitrogen spray cryotherapy in a single pig, spray cryotherapy produced the most evenly distributed lesion while complete separation of the squamous epithelium from underlying lamina propria was seen in all modalities, with the most extensive inflammation and necrosis in the muscularis seen with APC.[33] In another study, nine swine were treated with circumferential treatment in the distal esophagus using the liquid nitrogen system.[34] Dosimetry used was 5 seconds times four cycles (5 × 4), 5 seconds times six cycles (5 × 6), 10 seconds times four cycles (10 × 4), and 20 seconds times two cycles (20 × 2). In all groups, inflammation was seen into the

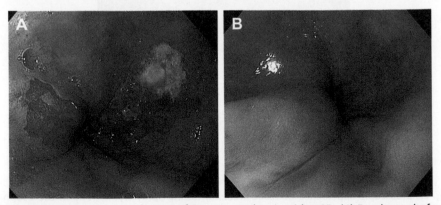

Fig. 3. Endoscopic spray cryotherapy of Barrett esophagus with HGD. (*A*) Esophagus before treatment. (*B*) Esophagus after cryotherapy treatment, with complete eradication of the intestinal metaplasia.

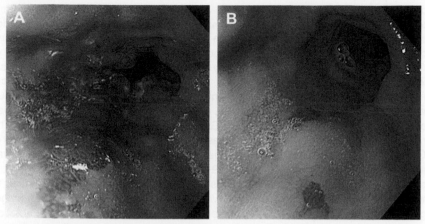

Fig. 4. Endoscopic spray cryotherapy in an 82-year-old woman with T1 submucosal adenocarcinoma who refused systemic therapy. (A) Narrow-band image of the midesophagus. Tumor is red-brown. (B) Narrow-band image of the esophagus after cryotherapy treatment, with complete eradication of the tumor and small residual areas of intestinal metaplasia.

muscularis propria with moderate to severe degree injury. In the 10 × 4 group, mean depth of injury was 4.75 mm with extension of necrosis into the submucosa in all animals and muscularis propria in some. In the 20 × 2 group, mean depth of injury was 5.3 mm with extension of necrosis into the submucosa only. In a separate study, eight swine were treated with varying duration of cryotherapy using the CO_2 system.[32] Depth of necrosis was proportional to duration of spray. Treatment for 15 seconds resulted in necrosis limited to the mucosa, while treatment for 30 seconds produced injury extending into the submucosa. Treatment for 45 and 60 seconds produced necrosis into the muscularis propria while 120-second treatment caused transmural necrosis. A human dosimetry study using the liquid nitrogen system is ongoing.

RESULTS OF TREATMENT
Barrett Esophagus With and Without Dysplasia

In 2005, Johnston and colleagues[35] presented their results using spray cryotherapy in the human esophagus. In this prospective single-center study, 11 patients with Barrett esophagus and varying degrees of dysplasia received hemicircumferential treatment at monthly intervals until the entire Barrett segment was eliminated. Mean Barrett segment length was 4.6 cm (range 1–8 cm). As for histology, 3 patients had Barrett esophagus without dysplasia, 2 were indefinite for dysplasia, 5 had low-grade dysplasia, and 1 had HGD. Complete endoscopic and histologic reversal of Barrett esophagus was seen in 9 of 11 patients treated (82%), although recurrent specialized intestinal metaplasia was seen at 6 months at the squamocolumnar junction in 2, yielding a success rate of 64% using an intention-to-treat analysis. No complications were reported, and all patients were free of subsquamous specialized intestinal metaplasia at 6-month follow-up. In 2006, these same investigators reported that circumferential spray (n = 10) was similar in efficacy to hemicircumferential therapy (n = 10) and required fewer treatment sessions (2.1 versus 4.8) to eradicate specialized intestinal metaplasia without increased formation of esophageal strictures.[36]

Dumot and colleagues[37] expanded on previous findings by treating 30 high-risk patients with HGD or IMCA who were deemed inoperable or who refused esophagectomy. These were considered challenging patients for ablation, with 8 receiving prior ablation (2 APC, 2 PDT, 3 endoscopic resection, and 1 PDT and endoscopic resection), including 1 patient with 10 cm of multifocal HGD after PDT and another with residual HGD at the esophagogastric junction after several sessions of PDT. Patients underwent serial cryotherapy sessions at 6-week intervals until mucosal disease resolved or progression was seen. Mean Barrett segment length was 6.1 cm (range 1–15 cm), mean number of treatment sessions was five, and median follow-up after treatment was 12 months. Response, defined as downgrading of histology, was seen in 27 of 30 (90%), including 92% of HGD patients and 80% of IMCA patients. The complete response for dysplasia (CR-D) was seen in 32% of HGD patients and 40% of IMCA patients. At 1 year, 78.1% of patients were cancer-free. Retreatment was needed in 11 patients (36.7%), including 9 of 26 with HGD and 2 of 5 with IMCA at baseline because of recurrence of dysplasia. Comparison of results of this study to other ablation studies is problematic. Many patients in this cohort had longer segments of Barrett esophagus and had failed other treatments, while most ablation trials enrolled only treatment-naïve patients with limited segment length disease.

One serious adverse event occurred in this study: A gastric rent caused by gastric distension from expanding nitrogen gas led to perforation in a patient with Marfan syndrome. This required surgical repair, and no further cryotherapy was given to this patient. Minor adverse events included chest pain occasionally requiring narcotic analgesics, mild stricture in three (all with narrowing from prior therapy before treatment), and lip ulcer in one. Most patients returned to their usual daily activities on the day following therapy.

In a safety and efficacy study from four centers of 77 patients treated with spray cryotherapy, efficacy data were presented in 23,[38] including 17 with HGD, 4 with IMCA, and 3 with early-stage adenocarcinoma. Complete response to HGD (CR-HGD) was seen in 94% with HGD and 100% with IMCA and cancer. Complete response to intestinal metaplasia (CR-IM) was seen in 53% with HGD, 75% with IMCA, and 67% with cancer. Mean follow-up in this study was 9.3 to 13.8 months. In the overall cohort, mean length of Barrett esophagus was 4 ± 3.6 cm, and the median number of treatments was four (range 1–10).

Results of a multicenter retrospective study assessing the safety and efficacy of cryotherapy in patients with HGD were recently presented.[39] Ninety-eight subjects were treated at 10 centers, and 61 patients completed therapy. The mean length of Barrett esophagus was 5 ± 3.2 cm, mean number of treatments was four, and median follow-up was 10.5 months. Endoscopic resection had been performed in 29.4% of the entire cohort before cryotherapy. Success rates for treatment were 97% for CR-HGD, 86% for CR-D, and 58% for CR-IM. In 275 follow-up biopsy sessions, 4 (1.5%) demonstrated subepithelial intestinal metaplasia ("buried Barrett").

Preliminary results on the success of CO_2 cryotherapy also have been presented recently.[40] Forty-four patients were treated, with mean Barrett segment length 4.8 cm, mean number of sessions was six (range 1–10), and median follow-up was 11.8 months (range 1–39). Nineteen patients were treatment naïve, while 18 had positive margin after endoscopic resection and 7 failed PDT or RFA. In the 22 patients who completed treatment, results include 91.3% CR-HGD, 95.6% CR-D, and 95.6% CR-IM. Adverse events were rare, with 2 patients reporting transient mild discomfort after therapy.

Esophageal Cancer

In 2007, the first use of spray cryotherapy for an esophageal neoplasm was published.[41] This 73-year-old man developed recurrent esophageal squamous cell carcinoma at the site of a previous squamous cell cancer treated with combination chemotherapy and radiation. Liquid nitrogen spray cryotherapy was used in two sessions. At the initial setting, dosimetry was 30 seconds times two freezes. At 1-month follow-up, the tumor had resolved endoscopically but persisted on biopsy. Repeat cryotherapy was performed for 20 seconds times three freezes. Although a significant stricture developed after this treatment, the patient remained cancer-free for 2 years. That same year, a series of four patients with T1/T2 esophageal cancer treated with cryotherapy was presented.[42] Each patient had failed or refused conventional treatment. Patients underwent treatment sessions every 3 to 6 weeks, with 4.3 mean treatments delivered over 3 to 11 months. Two patients had complete tumor regression at 6-week follow-up endoscopies after their last cryotherapy session and the other two demonstrated a greater than 50% reduction in the original tumor size.

Based on these encouraging but preliminary results, centers began using spray cryotherapy in patients who failed, refused, or were ineligible for conventional therapies, including surgery, chemotherapy, or radiation therapy. Results were collected and presented recently as a multicenter retrospective study.[43] Seventy-nine patients were enrolled; 74 had adenocarcinoma, and mean tumor length was 3.7 ± 3.5 cm. Tumor stage was T1 for 60 patients, T2 for 16 patients, T3 for 2 patients, and T4 for 1 patient. Forty-four patients completed therapy, either through complete tumor regression, progression of disease, or comorbid conditions. Complete eradication of tumor was seen in 31 of 44 patients (70.5%). In this group, final histology was normal squamous mucosa in 16 patients (51.6%), intestinal metaplasia in 10 patients (32.3%), low-grade dysplasia in 4 patients (12.9%), and HGD in 1 patient (3.2%). Median follow-up in this group was 15 months. Success of treatment by tumor stage was 77% (27 of 35) for T1, 60% (3 of 5) for T2, 50% (1 of 2) for T3, and 0% (0 of 1) for T4. Adverse events included stricture in 11 patients (15.1%) and postprocedure pain requiring narcotics in 20 (27%).

A recent report highlights the hemostatic effect of cryotherapy.[44] A 62-year-old man presented with an unresectable 10-cm hemorrhagic adenocarcinoma in the esophagus. He required 30 units of packed red blood cells over a 2-week period despite treatment with APC. The mass was treated with two cycles of 30-second spray with successful hemostasis, and the patient required only 1 additional unit of blood over the subsequent month until he expired.

Safety Profile

Patient comfort and safety are important considerations when choosing an ablation modality. PDT, the best-studied ablation modality for HGD, is associated with significant adverse events, including chest pain, nausea, vomiting, prolonged photosensitivity, and esophageal stricture.[14] A recent report compared symptoms in patients treated with PDT, RFA, and cryotherapy.[45] Fewer patients completing cryotherapy and RFA reported symptoms compared with those completing PDT. The investigators prospectively collected data on treatment-associated symptoms from 10 patients undergoing each treatment modality. Dysphagia and mild chest pain were the most common symptoms attributed to cryotherapy. RFA was associated with odynophagia, chest pain, and weight loss. PDT was associated with weight loss, chest pain, dysphagia/odynophagia, and phototoxicity. Esophageal strictures, requiring a single esophageal dilation, occurred in 1 patient having RFA and 2 patients with PDT.

A recent multicentered study presented findings from the largest to date collection of data on the safety and efficacy of endoscopic cryotherapy in 77 patients.[38] The study included 45 patients with HGD, 13 with IMCA, 10 with invasive cancer, 7 with nondysplastic Barrett esophagus, and 2 with severe squamous dysplasia. Each patient was contacted 1 to 10 days after each treatment session to gather data on side effects. Twenty-two patients (28%) were asymptomatic following all cryotherapy treatment sessions. In 323 total procedures, 168 (50%) were associated with symptoms. The most common complaint was chest pain (28.6%), dysphagia (17.6%), odynophagia (12.1%), and sore throat (9.6%). Symptoms were rated as mild in the majority of cases, and mean duration of symptoms was 3.6 ± 2.2 days. Symptoms were more likely in patients with segments of intestinal metaplasia 6 cm or longer. The previously noted patient with gastric perforation associated with Marfan syndrome was reported. Three esophageal strictures (4%) were reported in areas previously narrowed by peptic stricture or esophageal treatment. All were treated successfully by endoscopic dilation.

FUTURE DIRECTIONS

The results seen in the reported studies point to a promising future for endoscopic spray cryotherapy. Advances in treatment will likely occur through refinements in technique and technical improvements in equipment. Broader and better understanding of appropriate dosimetry for dysplasia and cancer will be gained with the completion of ongoing human studies. Adjuvant treatment with chemotherapy or radiation may augment the effects of cryotherapy in cancers and could further increase the success of treatment in esophageal cancer.

Extensive improvements in the low-pressure liquid-nitrogen device by CSA Medical are planned. A new device, scheduled to be available in 2010, contains multiple improvements. The ability to vary the flow rate of liquid nitrogen and integrated suction within the console will better address issues related to gastric distension during treatment. A new more flexible catheter design will enable better scope-tip manipulation and the ability to spray in the retroflexed position. Other improvements include reduced size (with a footprint half the size of the current system) and an updated control panel, which will enable custom dosimetry programs. Future improvements in the catheters and consoles should decrease frosting of the endoscope lens during treatment and enable treatment of larger areas of the esophagus in less time.

SUMMARY

Accumulating evidence highlights the promising results seen with endoscopic spray cryotherapy in the treatment of dysplasia associated with Barrett esophagus and esophageal carcinoma. Published studies show that the success of spray cryotherapy to eradicate Barrett high-grade dysplasia is comparable to that for other therapies, with a favorable safety profile and high levels of patient comfort. For patients with untreatable esophageal cancer, spray cryotherapy offers a therapeutic option with the potential for complete eradication in early-stage disease and palliation in advanced cases. The mechanism of tissue injury in cryotherapy is unique, with direct cytotoxic effects and ischemic effects from vascular injury. Increased tumor cell death through induction of apoptosis and immunologic effects require further study.

REFERENCES

1. Spechler SJ, Goyal RK. Barrett's esophagus. N Engl J Med 1986;315(6):362–71.
2. Champion G, Richter JE, Vaezi MF, et al. Duodenogastroesophageal reflux: relationship to pH and importance in Barrett's esophagus. Gastroenterology 1994; 107(3):747–54.

3. Eisen GM, Sandler RS, Murray S, et al. The relationship between gastroesopha-geal reflux disease and its complications with Barrett's esophagus. Am J Gastro-enterol 1997;92(1):27–31.
4. Reid BJ, Sanchez CA, Blount PL, et al. Barrett's esophagus: cell cycle abnormal-ities in advancing stages of neoplastic progression. Gastroenterology 1993; 105(1):119–29.
5. Stein HJ, Siewert JR. Barrett's esophagus: pathogenesis, epidemiology, func-tional abnormalities, malignant degeneration, and surgical management. Dysphagia 1993;8(3):276–88.
6. Devesa SS, Blot WJ, Fraumeni JF Jr. Changing patterns in the incidence of esophageal and gastric carcinoma in the United States. Cancer 1998;83(10): 2049–53.
7. Blot WJ, Devesa SS, Fraumeni JF Jr. Continuing climb in rates of esophageal adenocarcinoma: an update. JAMA 1993;270(11):1320.
8. Jemal A, Siegel R, Ward E, et al. Cancer statistics, 2008. CA Cancer J Clin 2008; 58(2):71–96.
9. Ries LAG, Melbert D, Krapcho M, et al, editors. SEER cancer statistics review. 1975–2004. Bethesda (MD): National Cancer Institute; Available at: http://seer. cancer.gov/csr/1975-2004/, based on November 2006 SEER data submission, posted to the SEER Web site, 2007. Accessed on May 15, 2009.
10. Rastogi A, Puli S, El-Serag HB, et al. Incidence of esophageal adenocarcinoma in patients with Barrett's esophagus and high-grade dysplasia: a meta-analysis. Gastrointest Endosc 2008;67(3):394–8.
11. Posner MC, Forastiere AA, Minsky BD. Cancer of the esophagus. In: Devita V, Hellman S, Rosenberg SA, editors. Cancer: principles & practice of oncology. 7th edition. Philadelphia: Lippincott Williams & Wilkins; 2005. p. 861–909.
12. Tadiparthi R, Bansal A, Sharma P. What's new in columnar lined esophagus (Bar-rett's metaplasia)? Curr Opin Gastroenterol 2008;24(4):516–20.
13. Pech O, Behrens A, May A, et al. Long-term results and risk factor analysis for recurrence after curative endoscopic therapy in 349 patients with high-grade in-traepithelial neoplasia and mucosal adenocarcinoma in Barrett's oesophagus. Gut 2008;57(9):1200–6.
14. Overholt BF, Lightdale CJ, Wang KK, et al. Photodynamic therapy with porfimer sodium for ablation of high-grade dysplasia in Barrett's esophagus: international, partially blinded, randomized phase III trial. Gastrointest Endosc 2005;62(4): 488–98.
15. Overholt BF, Panjehpour M, Halberg DL. Photodynamic therapy for Barrett's esophagus with dysplasia and/or early stage carcinoma: long-term results. Gas-trointest Endosc 2003;58(2):183–8.
16. Van Laethem JL, Jagodzinski R, Peny MO, et al. Argon plasma coagulation in the treatment of Barrett's high-grade dysplasia and in situ adenocarcinoma. Endos-copy 2001;33(3):257–61.
17. Shand A, Dallal H, Palmer K, et al. Adenocarcinoma arising in columnar lined oesophagus following treatment with argon plasma coagulation. Gut 2001; 48(4):580–1.
18. Sharma P, Jaffe PE, Bhattacharyya A, et al. Laser and multipolar electrocoagula-tion ablation of early Barrett's adenocarcinoma: long-term follow-up. Gastrointest Endosc 1999;49(4 Pt 1):442–6.
19. Sampliner RE, Fennerty B, Garewal HS. Reversal of Barrett's esophagus with acid suppression and multipolar electrocoagulation: preliminary results. Gastrointest Endosc 1996;44(5):532–5.

20. Ganz RA, Overholt BF, Sharma VK, et al. Circumferential ablation of Barrett's esophagus that contains high-grade dysplasia: a U.S. multicenter registry. Gastrointest Endosc 2008;68(1):35–40.
21. Shaheen NJ, Sharma P, Overholt BF, et al. Radiofrequency ablation in Barrett's esophagus with dysplasia. N Engl J Med 2009;360(22):2277–88.
22. Gage AA, Baust J. Mechanisms of tissue injury in cryosurgery. Cryobiology 1998; 37(3):171–86.
23. Baust JG, Gage AA. The molecular basis of cryosurgery. BJU Int 2005;95(9): 1187–91.
24. Kuflick E. Cryosurgery for cutaneous surgery—an update. Dermatol Surg 1997; 23(11):1081–7.
25. Wynn TA. Common and unique mechanisms regulate fibrosis in various fibroproliferative diseases. J Clin Invest 2007;117(3):524–9.
26. Hollister WR, Mathew AJ, Baust JG, et al. Effects of freezing on cell viability and mechanisms of cell death in a human prostate cell line. Mol Urol 1998;2(1):3–18.
27. Yang WL, Addona T, Nair DG, et al. Apoptosis induced by cryo-injury in human colorectal cancer cells is associated with mitochondrial dysfunction. Int J Cancer 2003;103(3):360–9.
28. Kwong KF. Molecular biology of esophageal cancer in the genomics era. Surg Clin North Am 2005;85(3):539–53.
29. Orlando RC. Pathogenesis of reflux esophagitis and Barrett's esophagus. Med Clin North Am 2005;89(2):219–41, vii.
30. Ablin RJ. An immune response: a possible caveat to endoscopic cryotherapy. Gastrointest Endosc 2001;53(7):840.
31. Dawber R. Cryosurgery: unapproved uses, dosages or indications. Clin Dermatol 2002;20(5):563–70.
32. Raju GS, Ahmed I, Xiao SY, et al. Graded esophageal mucosal ablation with cryotherapy, and the protective effects of submucosal saline. Endoscopy 2005;37(6): 523–6.
33. Eastone JA, Horwhat JD, Haluska O, et al. Cryoablation of swine esophageal mucosa: a direct comparison to argon plasma coagulation (APC) and multipolar electrocoagulation (MPEC) [abstract]. Gastrointest Endosc 2001;53:A3448.
34. Johnston L, Johnston MH. Cryospray ablation (CSA) in the esophagus: optimization of dosimetry [abstract]. Am J Gastroenterol 2006;101:S532.
35. Johnston MH, Eastone JA, Horwhat JD, et al. Cryoablation of Barrett's esophagus: a pilot study. Gastrointest Endosc 2005;62(6):842–8.
36. Johnston MH, Cash BD, Horwhat JD, et al. Cryoablation of Barrett's Esophagus (BE) [abstract]. Gastrointest Endosc 2006;130(4 Suppl 2):A640.
37. Dumot JA, Vargo JJ, Falk GW, et al. An open-label, prospective trial of cryospray ablation for Barrett's esophagus high-grade dysplasia and early esophageal cancer in high-risk patients. Gastrointest Endosc 2009 [Epub ahead of print].
38. Greenwald BD, Dumot JA, Horwhat JD, et al. Safety, tolerability, and efficacy of endoscopic low-pressure liquid nitrogen spray cryotherapy in the esophagus. Dis Esophagus 2009 [Epub ahead of print].
39. Shaheen NJ, Greenwald BD, Dumot JA, et al. Safety and efficacy of endoscopic spray cryotherapy for Barrett's esophagus with high-grade dysplasia [abstract]. Gastrointest Endosc 2009;69(5):AB357.
40. Canto MI, Gorospe EC, Shin EJ, et al. Carbon dioxide (CO_2) cryotherapy is a safe and effective treatment of Barrett's esophagus (BE) with HGD/intramucosal carcinoma [abstract]. Gastrointest Endosc 2009;69(5):AB341.

41. Cash BD, Johnston LR, Johnston MH. Cryospray ablation (CSA) in the palliative treatment of squamous cell carcinoma of the esophagus. World J Surg Oncol 2007;5:34–9.
42. Greenwald BD, Cash BD. Cryotherapy ablation of early stage esophageal cancer [abstract]. Gastrointest Endosc 2007;65(5):AB276.
43. Greenwald BD, Dumot JA, Abrams JA, et al. Endoscopic spray cryotherapy for esophageal cancer: safety and efficacy [abstract]. Gastrointest Endosc 2009; 69(5):AB349.
44. Schnoll-Sussman F. Cryospray ablation in the treatment of hemorrhagic esophageal cancer [abstract]. Am J Gastroenterol 2008;103(S1):S362.
45. Gross SA, Gill KR, Greenwald BD, et al. Burn, freeze or photo-ablate? Comparative symptom profile in patients with Barrett's high grade dysplasia undergoing endoscopic ablation [abstract]. Gastrointest Endosc 2008;67(5):AB180–1.

Recent Advances in Endoscopic Antireflux Techniques

Melina C. Vassiliou, MD, Med[a], Daniel von Renteln, MD[b],
Richard I. Rothstein, MD[c],*

KEYWORDS

• Gastroesophageal reflux disease
• Endoscopic antireflux therapy • Plication

GASTROESOPHAGEAL REFLUX DISEASE

Gastroesophageal reflux disease (GERD) has been defined as a condition that develops when reflux of stomach contents causes troublesome symptoms or complications.[1] The physiologic antireflux barrier is dependent on many factors, including lower esophageal sphincter (LES) complex, anatomy of the angle of His, and gastric distension. Pathologic reflux is associated with a decrease in LES pressure or obliteration of the angle of His.[2–4] The characteristic symptoms of GERD are retrosternal burning (pyrosis) and regurgitation.[1] GERD is common, but its prevalence varies geographically.[1,5,6] The prevalence of heartburn in a randomly selected adult population is approximately 10% to 20% in North America and Western Europe.[1,7–9] Esophageal erosions (reflux esophagitis) are the most common structural manifestations of the esophageal exposure to gastric acid. In a large study, including 194,527 patients with GERD, 45.4% had erosive esophagitis.[10] Other less common complications of GERD include ulceration (6.0%) or stricture formation (8.4%).[10] Barrett's esophagus can arise secondary to GERD, and esophageal intestinal metaplasia is the most important risk factor for esophageal adenocarcinoma. A study by Lagergren and colleagues demonstrated that risk of esophageal adenocarcinoma is increased for patients with GERD by an odds ratio of 7.7.[11]

MEDICAL THERAPY

Medical management of GERD using proton pump inhibitor (PPI) therapy is largely effective and considered standard therapy in treating symptoms and healing

[a] Department of Surgery, McGill University Health Centre, Montreal General Hospital, 1650 Cedar Avenue, L9-518, Montreal, Quebec, Canada H3G 1A4
[b] Department of Gastroenterology, Medizinische Klinik I, Klinikum Ludwigsburg, 71640 Ludwigsburg, Germany
[c] Section of Gastroenterology and Hepatology, Dartmouth-Hitchcock Medical Center, One Medical Center Drive, 4C, Lebanon, NH 03756, USA
* Corresponding author.
E-mail address: richard.rothstein@dartmouth.edu (R.I. Rothstein).

Gastrointest Endoscopy Clin N Am 20 (2010) 89–101
doi:10.1016/j.giec.2009.08.002
1052-5157/09/$ – see front matter © 2010 Elsevier Inc. All rights reserved.

esophagitis. A recent meta-analysis included 134 trials involving 35,978 patients and evaluated outcomes for treatment of esophagitis.[12] Five randomized controlled trials (RCTs) demonstrated a significant benefit from standard-dose PPI therapy compared with placebo. Ten RCTs reported a statistically significant benefit from H2-receptor antagonist (H2RA) compared with placebo. Three RCTs did not reveal any benefit from prokinetic therapy compared with placebo. Twenty six RCTs found PPIs superior to H2RA or H2RA plus prokinetics.[12] These acid-suppressing medications, although effective in controlling common reflux symptoms in the majority of patients with GERD, are often required indefinitely and can occasionally be associated with intolerable side effects and persistence of nonacid regurgitation.[4,12,13]

INTERVENTIONAL THERAPY

Interventional therapies for GERD include surgical or endoscopic techniques. All interventional therapies need to consider the pathophysiology of GERD and the anatomy of the gastroesophageal (GE) junction. Interventional therapy, therefore, should aim to alter the GE junction anatomy to prevent transient LES relaxation, increase baseline LES tone, or increase baseline LES length.

PATIENT PRETHERAPEUTIC ASSESSMENT

Response rates of up to 50% have been reported for GERD with placebo therapy. As such, meticulous pre- and post-therapeutic assessment, which allows for objective measurement of GERD, is essential.[14] An upper gastrointestinal endoscopy should be performed at baseline before endoscopic therapy for GERD to determine presence and size of a hiatal hernia, grade the degree of esophagitis, and determine if contraindications to endoscopic therapy are present. In patients with hiatal hernias greater than 3 cm, surgical treatment is recommended and preferred over endoscopic therapy. Most initial studies investigating endoscopic antireflux therapies excluded patients with grade IV esophagitis, Barrett's epithelium, persistent dysphagia, or esophageal strictures.[15–22]

Successful outcome of antireflux surgery can be predicted by an abnormal 24-hour pH test, the presence of typical reflux symptoms, and a favorable response to acid suppression therapy.[23] Accordingly, patients being considered for endoscopic antireflux therapy should have symptomatic relief from PPI therapy and pathologic acid exposure defined as having distal esophageal pH less than 4.0 for at least 4.5% of a 24- or 48-hour monitoring period or a DeMeester score greater than or equal to 14.7. A limitation of traditional pH monitoring is that only reflux episodes with a pH drop below 4 are detected. Symptomatic nonacidic reflux or regurgitation of gastric contents neutralized by food or antisecretory therapy cannot be detected by this technique. Because the pH probe measures acid concentration regularly at a single pH sensor, it also cannot determine bolus volume, transit, or composition or localize the reflux within the esophagus. Multichannel intraluminal impedance monitoring (MII) is a relatively novel method, which addresses these limitations by reporting esophageal bolus transit in addition to pH data. Detection of nonacid or weakly acidic reflux events, aerophagia, and differentiation of true reflux events from nonreflux events (acidic or nonacidic swallows) is possible with MII monitoring.[13,24–30] MII assessment before and after endoscopic antireflux therapy seems ideal to document objective changes in reflux events. Recent studies have shown MII a useful tool in selecting patients for antireflux surgery. Patients with a positive symptom index resistant to PPIs with nonacid or acid reflux demonstrated by MII monitoring proved good candidates for laparoscopic Nissen fundoplication.[25,26,28,31]

SURGICAL THERAPY

As a therapeutic alternative to PPI treatment, laparoscopic Nissen fundoplication is considered safe and effective, especially for patients with significantly sized hiatal hernias. A recent meta-analysis, including 12 RCTs, compared laparoscopic and open antireflux surgery for the treatment of proved GERD.[32] The meta-analysis demonstrated a significant reduction in the duration of hospital stay (2.68 days) and a significant reduction in time for return to normal activity (7.75 days), favoring the laparoscopic group. There was a statistically significant reduction of 65% in the relative odds of complication rates for the laparoscopic group. Treatment failure rates were comparable between both groups. On the basis of this meta-analysis, the investigators concluded that laparoscopic treatment is as effective but safer than open surgical treatment for GERD.[32] Both surgical approaches are associated with significant complications and side effects, and a significant minority of patients undergoing fundoplication may need to return to medication use to control symptoms over time.

ENDOSCOPIC ANTIREFLUX TECHNIQUES

Several endoscopic antireflux procedures have been evaluated for the treatment of GERD. These techniques (**Table 1**) include the injection or implantation of biopolymers, the application of radiofrequency energy to the LES, and endoluminal suturing/plication.[15–22,33–39] Endoscopic treatment strategies currently target PPI-dependent GERD patients with small (<3 cm) or absent hiatal hernias who do not have severe esophagitis or Barrett's esophagus. Thus far, EndoCinch (BARD, Billerica, Massachusetts), Enteryx (Boston Scientific, Natick, Massachusetts), Stretta (Curon Medical, Sunnyvale, California), and the Plicator (NDO Surgical, Mansfield, Massachusetts) have been studied in sham-controlled trials (see **Table 1**).[17,40–43]

Enteryx

Enteryx is a biocompatible polymer consisting of 8% ethylene vinyl alcohol mixed with tantalum powder that provided for radiographic opacification, in a solution of dimethyl sulfoxide. It is liquid before injection and becomes an inert spongy mass once injected into tissue. The procedure requires a special 4-mm, 23-gauge injector needle and the use of fluoroscopy. The standard procedure was placement of 1 mL or more of volume circumferentially around the GE junction until approximately 6 to 8 mL of Enteryx was implanted intramuscularly. The Enteryx procedure was repeatable if symptom control was inadequate but not reversible. Enteryx is no longer marketed or available for human clinical use.

Table 1		
Endoscopic antireflux techniques		
Injection or Implantation	Thermal Energy	Endoscopic Suturing, Plicating, or Stapling
Enteryx	Stretta (radiofrequency ablation)	Wilson-Cook ESD
Gatekeeper		EndoCinch
Durasphere		Plicator
		EsophyX
		Syntheon Anti-Reflux Device
		His-Wiz antireflux device
		Medigus SRS

An international multicenter study of 85 patients treated with Enteryx demonstrated cessation of PPI use in 74% of treated subjects at 6 months and, at 12-month follow-up, 70% of these subjects had significant improvements in objective measure of acid reflux (pH scores). pH normalization was encountered in 38.8% of patients at 12 months and the LES was approximately 1 cm longer after therapy. In the treated cohort, there was no effect on the incidence or severity of esophagitis after treatment. The GERD–*health-related quality-of-life* (HRQL) scores after Enteryx were comparable with those obtained on antisecretory medications. Complications included chest pain (92%) that resolved within l4 days in 83% of affected individuals and dysphagia (20%) that resolved within 2 to 12 weeks. There was one death related to Enteryx injection into the aortic wall that led to withdrawal of the device from the market.[44,45]

Gatekeeper

The Gatekeeper Reflux Repair System (Medtronic, Minneapolis, Minnesota) restricts the diameter of the distal esophagus by submucosal implantation of a polyacrylonitrile-based hydrogel prosthesis. The device consists of a 16-mm overtube-type instrument through which a standard or pediatric-sized videogastroscope was passed, to monitor the procedure. Suction was used to draw mucosal tissue into multiple, shallow holes in the distal part of the Gatekeeper instrument and to place the hydrogel prostheses submucosally. A 1-mm diameter flexible endoscopic injector needle and a 1-mm trocar needle catheter were used through another channel in the overtube to prepare the submucosal region for implantation of the prosthesis. Usually, four to six implants were placed in a radial fashion during one treatment session. This implantation technique was repeatable and reversible.

A pilot study included 10 GERD patients and demonstrated successful implant placement in 97% of attempts. The procedures improved reflux symptom scores at 1 and 6 months' follow-up. Four of 9 patients stopped their acid-suppressing medicines, whereas three reduced their PPI dosage by at least 50%.[46] Pooled data from two prospective nonrandomized trials reported data for 68 patients treated with this method. At 6 months, time with pH less than 4 improved from 9.1% to 6.1% (n = 45, $P<.05$), LES pressure was slightly higher, and GERD-HRQL scores went from 24 to 5 ($P<.01$). Two adverse events occurred: one patient suffered a pharyngeal perforation, and severe postprandial nausea was reported in another patient that resolved after endoscopic removal of the prostheses.[47] An international, multicenter, sham-controlled trial was started for this device but was subsequently cancelled before completion, and the device is no longer available.

Durasphere

Durasphere (Carbon Medical Technologies, St Paul, Minnesota) is a Food and Drug Administration–approved injectable agent that has been used to treat urinary incontinence since 1999. It consists of carbon-coated beads ranging from 90 to 212 μm suspended in a water-based gel. The particles were specifically designed to prevent migration and are inert. This agent was recently used to treat 10 patients with objectively proved GERD on PPI therapy. The substance was injected submucosally at the Z-line in four quadrants using a standard endoscopic sclerotherapy needle. The patients were followed for 12 months and five of them were retreated within 90 days for poor symptom control. At the end of the study, the patients were found to have a significant reduction in DeMeester scores from 44.5 to 26.5. Four of the 9 patients followed had normal pH testing. The material and bulk effect was still in place at endoscopy 1 year later and adverse events, such as substernal pain and difficulty belching, were minor and transient.[48] Further data are needed, including a randomized, controlled trial, but these initial results demonstrate a straightforward, safe technique with measurable symptom improvement.

RADIOFREQUENCY ABLATION

The Stretta System delivers low-power, temperature-controlled radiofrequency energy to the GE junction. The system consists of a special 20-French, balloon-basket, single-use catheter with four radially distributed, curved, 25-gauge, 5.5-mm long, nickel-titanium needles. Each needle is equipped with dual thermocouple temperature sensors to maintain consistent energy delivery to the muscular layer. Ports in the catheter provide cold-water irrigation during the procedure to reduce mucosal heating and prevent surface tissue injury. The radiofrequency generator is a computerized control module unit that delivers the radiofrequency energy to the needle electrodes. The target temperature for tissue thermal treatment was 85 °C. The full Stretta procedure involves applying thermal radiofrequency treatment in four antegrade rings that straddle the GE junction from 1 cm above to just beneath the squamocolumnar junction in 0.5 cm increments. The irreversible procedure takes approximately 45 minutes.

A sham-controlled study of 64 GERD patients demonstrated Stretta treatment (performed in 35 patients) as superior to sham (in 29 patients) for control of heartburn symptoms and improvement in quality of life at 6 months after the intervention. Although there were more Stretta-treated than sham subjects who responded to the intervention (defined as >50% improvement in GERD quality-of-life score) at 6 months (61% vs 30%), and more treated than sham who were without daily heartburn symptoms at this follow-up interval (61% vs 33%), no differences in reduction of daily medication use were evident between the groups. There were also no differences in esophageal acid exposure times between the two groups at 6 months.[41] The Stretta System is no longer marketed or available for human clinical use.

SUTURING, PLICATING, OR STAPLING DEVICES
Wilson-Cook Endoscopic Suturing Device

The Endoscopic Suturing Device (ESD) (Cook Medical, Bloomington, Indiana) consists of an external accessory channel, a flexible Sew-Right device, and a flexible Ti-Knot device. The external accessory channel is attached to a flexible endoscope and provides the pathway for the Sew-Right and Ti-Knot devices. The flexible Sew-Right device is a dual-needle system that uses a single suture loop to create the tissue plication. The target tissue is aspirated into a suction chamber. A needle with suture is then passed through the tissue collected within the chamber. A continuous single suture loop is used to stitch two adjacent areas in the proximal stomach to form the plication. With the ESD, no repeated endoscope withdrawals are required to create the gastric plication. Typically, two or three plications are placed during a single treatment. The ESD is no longer marketed or available for human clinical use.

Studies revealed early loss of the sutures. At 6 months, only 5% of the sutures were found in situ. No significant changes in reflux esophagitis or 24-hour pH monitoring were observed at 6 months (median pH <4/24 h, 9.9% vs 12.3% [therapy vs baseline]; $P = .60$). LES sphincter pressure was unchanged (median LES pressure 7.2 mm Hg vs 9.9 mm Hg; $P = .22$). PPI use was not improved either.[18] A second uncontrolled study confirmed the same poor outcomes mainly related to early loss of the sutures.[37]

BARD EndoCinch

The EndoCinch suturing device is inserted via an overtube. A sewing capsule is attached to the distal tip of a standard videogastroscope and has a cavity into which a tissue fold can be suctioned. A handle is attached to the biopsy port of the endoscope and controls the advance of a hollow-core suturing needle. A treasury-tag (t-tag) is back-loaded into the hollow-bore needle and is captured into the tip of the capsule after being driven forward by a stiff wire pushed through the hollow needle. It can be reloaded and a second area of tissue can be captured. The two captured areas are drawn together to create a tissue plication. A catheter cuts the suture ends as it cinches together the tag components at the luminal surface. Stitches to form plications can be placed in a linear, circumferential, or helical fashion. Typically two or three plications are created at a treatment session.

A sham-controlled, randomized study available published as an abstract demonstrated improved heartburn frequency at 3 months' post treatment for the EndoCinch group (69% vs 31%, $P = .03$). There was no significant difference in heartburn severity (81% vs 50%), regurgitation (53% vs 56%), or bothersome scores (75% vs 50%). More subjects in the gastric plication group discontinued their daily acid-suppressing medications compared with sham treatment (75% vs 25%; $P = .01$). No difference was found comparing use of acid-suppressive medications (56% vs 25%), however. Acid exposure significantly improved in the EndoCinch versus sham groups (pH difference: -4.0 vs +1.0; $P = .03$) but normalized only in two (12.5%) treated patients. The study did not detect a difference between treated and sham patients on LES pressure or quality-of-life measures.[49]

An uncontrolled, single-center study, including 70 patients, demonstrated long-term treatment failure mainly due to suture loss. Eighteen months after treatment, 56 of 70 patients (80%) did not improve their heartburn symptoms or PPI medication use by greater than 50%. Endoscopy exhibited all sutures in situ in 12 of 70 (17%) patients and no remaining sutures in 18 of 70 (26%). In 54 and 50 patients examined, no significant changes in 24-hour pH monitoring (median pH <4/24 h, 9.1% vs 8.5%; $P = .82$) or LES pressure (7.7 vs 10.3 mm Hg; $P = .051$) were observed respectively, whereas median LES length increased slightly (3.0 to 3.2 cm; $P<.05$).[50]

A second sham-controlled study demonstrated reduced acid-inhibitory drug use and improved GERD symptoms and improved the quality of life at 3 months compared with a sham procedure. No difference in reduction of esophageal acid exposure was seen after endoscopic treatment compared with sham procedure. Due to suture loss, the effects only persisted up to 12 months.[19]

NDO Plicator

The NDO Plicator was designed to create a transmural full-thickness placation at the angle of His. The plication is formed with a pretied, suture-based implant. The Plicator can be advanced into the stomach over a Savary guide wire and is retroflexed for placement of the full-thickness sutures at the GE junction. Visualization is accomplished using a 5.9-mm flexible endoscope inserted through a dedicated channel in the instrument. This plicating device remodels the antireflux barrier at the angle of His by fashioning a pleat of full-thickness tissue and permitting serosa-to-serosa apposition. The components of the system include the plicator instrument, a tissue retracting helical catheter, and pretied pledgeted suture implants. The plicator has a handle with wheels for opening/closing the arms and sliding/locking the pretied suture implant. The total procedure time is approximately 10 to 20 minutes to form a single plication. Newer data suggest that placement of 2 to 3 implants may be preferable to optimally restructure the GE junction.[20–22]

A sham-controlled trial randomly assigned 159 patients to plication (n = 78) or a sham procedure (n = 81). The percentage reduction in esophageal pH time less than 4 was significantly improved in the plication group (7% vs 10% compared with baseline) but not in the sham group (10% vs 9%). There were no perforations or deaths. Four patients required hospitalization for postprocedure pain and one required exploratory laparoscopy 3 months after the procedure for persistent abdominal pain.[17] Recent studies have used serial implants to improve restructuring of the angle of His and demonstrated significant reductions in esophageal acid exposure, esophagitis, and PPI use at 6 and 12 months.[20–22] The NDO device is no longer available on for commercial use.

EsophyX

EsophyX (EndoGastric Solutions, Redmond, Washington) is a large overtube device with an insertion channel for a videogastroscope. It also includes a bending section, or elbow, which can articulate and retroflex to reach and manipulate tissue at the angle of His. The system is designed to create a 270° circumferential endoscopic plication at the angle of His. The technique uses a helical retractor to engage and manipulate tissue at the fundus and to create the correct angle. After tissue grasping and fixation, double-sided t-tags can be passed through a double layer full-thickness plication. The method involves the placement of approximately 6 to 14 sutures to create a near circumferential gastroplication of 180° to 260°. The device can be used to reduce small hiatal hernias. EsophyX is Conformite Europeenne marked and available in Europe and recently received Food and Drug Administration clearance in the United States.

No randomized controlled data are reported to date. Early clinical experience assessed the degree of postprocedural valve tightness relative to the gastroscope and reported the valves as tightly adherent in 14 and moderately adherent in 3 of 17 cases. The hiatal hernias present in 13 of 17 patients were all reduced. Adverse events reported include mild-to-moderate pharyngeal irritation and epigastric pain, which all resolved spontaneously. At 12-month follow-up (n = 16), the valve length had a mean of 3 cm (range 1 to 4 cm) and circumference of 200° (150° to 210°). Eighty-one percent of the valves retained their tightness. The hiatal hernias, present in 76% of subjects initially, were now found in 38%. The median GERD-HRQL scores improved by 67% and 9 of 17 patients (82%) were still off their PPI medications, whereas normalization of the pH was seen in 63%.[51,52] Recent 2-year data were published by the same group, which included 14 of the initial 19 patients. The long-term safety profile of the device is good, and it seems as though the restructured anatomy is durable when examined endoscopically. Among the patients treated, 29% were completely relieved of GERD, 60% of hiatal hernias were reduced, and esophagitis was eliminated in 55% of individuals.[53] This data must be interpreted with caution because they are essentially all from a single center, and a single, small cohort of patients. The only North American study using this device is a retrospective report of eight patients who underwent the procedure. Half of the patients did not benefit from the procedure, and one patient had clear disruption of the sutures. Two patients were off PPIs and the other two were on reduced doses of the medication.[54] Much further study is needed, including a prospective RCT.

Syntheon Anti-Reflux Device

Using this device, a titanium implant is delivered into the cardia to create a serosa-to-serosa apposition similar to the Plicator. The Anti-Reflux Device (Syntheon, Miami, FL) instrument differs from the Plicator in that the device can be passed alongside the endoscope and controlled independently. A catheter-based tissue retractor through the endoscope biopsy channel is used to pull the gastric wall into the jaws of the Anti-Reflux Device. The titanium implant is deployed as the jaws close, to create a full-thickness pleat. Results of a multicenter clinical trial have been published in abstract form. Seventy GERD patients were treated, and 57 had been followed for a minimum of 6 months at the time of abstract publication. GERD-HRQL improved by 50% or more in 79% of the subjects. At 6 months, 33 of 52 individuals (63%) stopped all antisecretory therapy. The implants were all found in place on follow-up endoscopy and one gastric perforation occurred requiring surgical repair.[55] Despite superior engineering, the Anti-Reflux Device was not brought forward to commercialization.

The His-Wiz Antireflux Procedure

Another overtube-based endoscopic suturing machine, coined the His-Wiz (Apollo Group/Olympus Optical, Tokyo, Japan), allows for full-thickness suturing and cutting in a single step. Two plications are performed, one anterior and the other posterior, just below the Z-line. A small clinical trial of seven patients with 1-year follow-up is available in abstract form. Subjective (heartburn scores) and objective (pH testing) improvements were observed, but the effect seemed to deteriorate slowly over time.[56] Based on these preliminary data, the durability and effectiveness of this procedure are still unknown, and the device has not been brought forward to commercialization.

The Medigus Endoscopy System

Few data are available regarding this novel device (Medigus SRS, Omer, Israel), which consists of an ultrasonic video endoscope and an integrated surgical stapler. The cartridge is mounted onto the shaft of the scope and the anvil is at the tip. B-shaped, 4.8-mm staples are fired under ultrasound guidance to create an anterior, full-thickness, 180° fundoplication. One Medigus-sponsored survival porcine study has been published to date using this device. Twelve animals successfully underwent the procedure and survived for 6 weeks. The mean procedure time was 12 minutes, and all of the fundoplications seemed to be in place at the end of the study.[57] More data will be available from a recently initiated international human clinical trial using this highly refined technology.

SUMMARY

The goal of GERD therapy is to control symptoms, heal esophageal mucosa, and prevent complications, such as Barrett's metaplasia. Pharmacologic therapy is effective for symptom relief, mucosal healing, and long-term maintenance of remission. The need for daily administration, failure to provide complete symptom relief, and possible side effects, however, may limit the use in some patients, prompting consideration of alternative treatment strategies. The idea of minimally invasive treatments, as an alternative to surgical intervention, stimulated the development of several endoscopic techniques for the treatment of GERD. Most of the available data on endoluminal GERD therapies, however, suggest that endoscopic interventions produce significant, but often short-term, improvements in GERD-related quality of life and reduction of antireflux medication intake. Despite symptomatic improvement in the majority of studies, acid exposure was not significantly reduced and LES pressure was not typically improved. Radiofrequency treatment (Stretta) seemed modestly effective but is currently unavailable. Implantation techniques have largely been abandoned due to lack of long-term efficacy (Gatekeeper) and serious side effects (Enteryx). Recently, the concept of injectable bulking agents for the treatment of GERD has been re-evaluated (Durasphere) and seems associated with symptomatic improvement in patients with mild to moderate GERD.[48]

First-generation endoluminal suturing techniques (EndoCinch and ESD) demonstrated a proof of principle but they lacked durability and long-term effectiveness. Therefore, the endoscopic plication technique (Plicator) was developed with the intention to place transmural sutures. A RCT suggested that endoscopic full-thickness plication is significantly better compared with sham treatment for control of GERD symptoms, use of antisecretory medication, and distal esophageal acid exposure. Three- and 5-year durability of the pledgeted sutures and the treatment effect (sustained symptom relief and decreased medication use) also has been demonstrated. The use of multiple Plicator implants, as opposed to a single implant placed in the initial trials, demonstrated significant improvement in reflux symptoms, esophagitis, medication use, and esophageal acid exposure. EsophyX is a similar device for endoluminal fundoplication that allows the placement of transmural implants. Published data are limited but suggest some improvement in GERD symptoms and medication use. RCTs are necessary to evaluate the safety and efficacy of this and other emerging techniques.

When considering the outcomes of all of these different methods, one must keep in mind that many of these techniques are associated with a substantial learning curve and that most of the published/presented data are collections of a few cases from different institutions that likely were still in their learning curve. Furthermore, for varying reasons, some promising and well-engineered therapies have become unavailable, making further data collection and investigation impossible. Certainly, as industry and clinicians partner together and continue to develop robust endoscopic devices for translumenal and natural orifice translumenal endoscopic (NOTES) surgery, some of these technologies may prove effective for creating intralumenal fundoplications resulting in effective and durable treatments. The ideal method needs to be practical, easy to perform, and reliable. Furthermore, although partial improvements in esophageal acid exposure may be achievable and helpful for treating symptoms, the ultimate effect on preventing GERD-related complications is unclear and is still a concern associated with all of these methods.

At this time, given the effectiveness and excellent outcomes of minimally invasive antireflux surgery and pharmacologic therapy, available E-ARTs cannot be recommended for routine clinical use, and endoscopic GERD treatment should be undertaken in institutional review board–approved clinical studies or in clinical application that includes entering the procedure and outcome data into a central registry. Randomized trials comparing endoscopic reflux therapies to medical or surgical therapy are necessary to better understand the value of endoscopic treatment and the ideal target population and to make evidence-based recommendations for patient care. Although at present there is no endoscopic reflux treatment for routine clinical application, a substantial gap still exists between antisecretory drugs and surgical therapy that might be bridged by means of safe and effective endoscopic therapies. The continued development of devices to provide safe, effective, and durable outcomes is expected but requires a collaboration of regulatory and reimbursement agencies working together with entrepreneurs and manufacturers to be successful.

REFERENCES

1. Vakil N, van Zanten SV, Kahrilas P, et al. The Montreal definition and classification of gastroesophageal reflux disease: a global evidence-based consensus. Am J Gastroenterol 2006;101:1900.
2. Hirsch DP, Mathus-Vliegen EM, Dagli U, et al. Effect of prolonged gastric distention on lower esophageal sphincter function and gastroesophageal reflux. Am J Gastroenterol 2003;98:1696.
3. Massey BT. Potential control of gastroesophageal reflux by local modulation of transient lower esophageal sphincter relaxations. Am J Med 2001;111(Suppl 8): 186S.
4. Tack J. Recent developments in the pathophysiology and therapy of gastroesophageal reflux disease and nonerosive reflux disease. Curr Opin Gastroenterol 2005; 21:454.
5. El-Serag H, Hill C, Jones R. Systematic review: the epidemiology of gastro-oesophageal reflux disease in primary care, using the UK General Practice Research Database. Aliment Pharmacol Ther 2009;29:470.
6. Fujimoto K. Review article: prevalence and epidemiology of gastro-oesophageal reflux disease in Japan. Aliment Pharmacol Ther 2004;20(Suppl 8):5.
7. Delaney BC. Review article: prevalence and epidemiology of gastro-oesophageal reflux disease. Aliment Pharmacol Ther 2004;20(Suppl 8):2.
8. Dent J, El-Serag HB, Wallander MA, et al. Epidemiology of gastro-oesophageal reflux disease: a systematic review. Gut 2005;54:710.
9. Spechler SJ. Epidemiology and natural history of gastro-oesophageal reflux disease. Digestion 1992;51(Suppl 1):24.
10. el-Serag HB, Sonnenberg A. Associations between different forms of gastro-oesophageal reflux disease. Gut 1997;41:594.
11. Lagergren J, Bergstrom R, Lindgren A, et al. Symptomatic gastroesophageal reflux as a risk factor for esophageal adenocarcinoma. N Engl J Med 1999; 340:825.
12. Khan M, Santana J, Donnellan C, et al. Medical treatments in the short term management of reflux oesophagitis. Cochrane Database Syst Rev 2007;(2):CD003244.
13. Mainie I, Tutuian R, Shay S, et al. Acid and non-acid reflux in patients with persistent symptoms despite acid suppressive therapy: a multicentre study using combined ambulatory impedance-pH monitoring. Gut 2006;55:1398.
14. Hogan WJ. Clinical trials evaluating endoscopic GERD treatments: is it time for a moratorium on the clinical use of these procedures? Am J Gastroenterol 2006;101:437.
15. Chen D, Barber C, McLoughlin P, et al. Systematic review of endoscopic treatments for gastro-oesophageal reflux disease. Br J Surg 2009;96:128.
16. Pleskow D, Rothstein R, Kozarek R, et al. Endoscopic full-thickness plication for the treatment of GERD: five-year long-term multicenter results. Surg Endosc 2008;22:326.
17. Rothstein R, Filipi C, Caca K, et al. Endoscopic full-thickness plication for the treatment of gastroesophageal reflux disease: a randomized, sham-controlled trial. Gastroenterology 2006;131:704.
18. Schiefke I, Neumann S, Zabel-Langhennig A, et al. Use of an endoscopic suturing device (the "ESD") to treat patients with gastroesophageal reflux disease, after unsuccessful EndoCinch endoluminal gastroplication: another failure. Endoscopy 2005;37:700.

19. Schwartz MP, Wellink H, Gooszen HG, et al. Endoscopic gastroplication for the treatment of gastro-oesophageal reflux disease: a randomised, sham-controlled trial. Gut 2007;56:20.
20. von Renteln D, Brey U, Riecken B, et al. Endoscopic full-thickness plication (Plicator) with two serially placed implants improves esophagitis and reduces PPI use and esophageal acid exposure. Endoscopy 2008;40:173.
21. von Renteln D, Schiefke I, Fuchs KH, et al. Endoscopic full-thickness plication for the treatment of gastroesophageal reflux disease using multiple Plicator implants: 12-month multicenter study results. Surg Endosc 2009;23(8):1866–75.
22. von Renteln D, Schiefke I, Fuchs KH, et al. Endoscopic full-thickness plication for the treatment of GERD by application of multiple Plicator implants: a multicenter study (with video). Gastrointest Endosc 2008;68:833.
23. Campos GM, Peters JH, DeMeester TR, et al. Multivariate analysis of factors predicting outcome after laparoscopic Nissen fundoplication. J Gastrointest Surg 1999;3:292.
24. Bredenoord AJ, Weusten BL, Timmer R, et al. Reproducibility of multichannel intraluminal electrical impedance monitoring of gastroesophageal reflux. Am J Gastroenterol 2005;100:265.
25. del Genio G, Tolone S, del Genio F, et al. Prospective assessment of patient selection for antireflux surgery by combined multichannel intraluminal impedance pH monitoring. J Gastrointest Surg 2008;12:1491.
26. del Genio G, Tolone S, del Genio F, et al. Total fundoplication controls acid and nonacid reflux: evaluation by pre- and postoperative 24-h pH-multichannel intraluminal impedance. Surg Endosc 2008;22:2518.
27. Ford CN. Evaluation and management of laryngopharyngeal reflux. JAMA 2005; 294:1534.
28. Gruebel C, Linke G, Tutuian R, et al. Prospective study examining the impact of multichannel intraluminal impedance on antireflux surgery. Surg Endosc 2008;22: 1241.
29. Tutuian R, Castell DO. Reflux monitoring: role of combined multichannel intraluminal impedance and pH. Gastrointest Endosc Clin N Am 2005;15:361.
30. Vela MF. Non-acid reflux: detection by multichannel intraluminal impedance and pH, clinical significance and management. Am J Gastroenterol 2009; 104:277.
31. Mainie I, Tutuian R, Agrawal A, et al. Combined multichannel intraluminal impedance-pH monitoring to select patients with persistent gastro-oesophageal reflux for laparoscopic Nissen fundoplication. Br J Surg 2006;93:1483.
32. Peters MJ, Mukhtar A, Yunus RM, et al. Meta-analysis of randomized clinical trials comparing open and laparoscopic anti-reflux surgery. Am J Gastroenterol 2009; 104:1548.
33. Chuttani R. Endoscopic full-thickness plication: the device, technique, pre-clinical and early clinical experience. Gastrointest Endosc Clin N Am 2003;13:109.
34. Dolan JP, Downey DM, Sheppard BC, et al. Evaluation of endoscopic full-thickness plication on anti-reflux valve competency. J Surg Educ 2008;65:140.
35. Filipi CJ, Lehman GA, Rothstein RI, et al. Transoral, flexible endoscopic suturing for treatment of GERD: a multicenter trial. Gastrointest Endosc 2001;53:416.
36. Rothstein RI. Endoscopic therapy of gastroesophageal reflux disease: outcomes of the randomized-controlled trials done to date. J Clin Gastroenterol 2008;42: 594.
37. Schilling D, Kiesslich R, Galle PR, et al. Endoluminal therapy of GERD with a new endoscopic suturing device. Gastrointest Endosc 2005;62:37.

38. Sgouros SN, Bergele C. Endoscopic therapy for gastroesophageal reflux disease: a systematic review. Digestion 2006;74:1.
39. Swain P, Park PO, Mills T. Bard EndoCinch: the device, the technique, and pre-clinical studies. Gastrointest Endosc Clin N Am 2003;13:75.
40. Comay D, Adam V, da Silveira EB, et al. The Stretta procedure versus proton pump inhibitors and laparoscopic Nissen fundoplication in the management of gastroesophageal reflux disease: a cost-effectiveness analysis. Can J Gastroenterol 2008;22:552.
41. Corley DA, Katz P, Wo JM, et al. Improvement of gastroesophageal reflux symptoms after radiofrequency energy: a randomized, sham-controlled trial. Gastroenterology 2003;125:668.
42. Deviere J, Costamagna G, Neuhaus H, et al. Nonresorbable copolymer implantation for gastroesophageal reflux disease: a randomized sham-controlled multicenter trial. Gastroenterology 2005;128:532.
43. Domagk D, Menzel J, Seidel M, et al. Endoluminal gastroplasty (EndoCinch) versus endoscopic polymer implantation (Enteryx) for treatment of gastroesophageal reflux disease: 6-month results of a prospective, randomized trial. Am J Gastroenterol 2006;101:422.
44. Johnson DA, Ganz R, Aisenberg J, et al. Endoscopic implantation of enteryx for treatment of GERD: 12-month results of a prospective, multicenter trial. Am J Gastroenterol 1921;98:2003.
45. Johnson DA, Ganz R, Aisenberg J, et al. Endoscopic, deep mural implantation of Enteryx for the treatment of GERD: 6-month follow-up of a multicenter trial. Am J Gastroenterol 2003;98:250.
46. Fockens P. Gatekeeper Reflux Repair System: technique, pre-clinical, and clinical experience. Gastrointest Endosc Clin N Am 2003;13:179.
47. Fockens P, Bruno MJ, Gabbrielli A, et al. Endoscopic augmentation of the lower esophageal sphincter for the treatment of gastroesophageal reflux disease: multicenter study of the gatekeeper reflux repair system. Endoscopy 2004;36:682.
48. Ganz RA, Fallon E, Wittchow T, et al. A new injectable agent for the treatment of GERD: results of the Durasphere pilot trial. Gastrointest Endosc 2009;69:318.
49. Rothstein RI, Hynes ML, Grove MR, et al. Endoscopic gastric plication (EndoCinch) for GERD: a randomized, sham-controlled, blinded, single-center study. Gastrointest Endosc 2004;59:P111.
50. Schiefke I, Zabel-Langhennig A, Neumann S, et al. Long term failure of endoscopic gastroplication (EndoCinch). Gut 2005;54:752.
51. Cadiere GB, Rajan A, Germay O, et al. Endoluminal fundoplication by a transoral device for the treatment of GERD: a feasibility study. Surg Endosc 2008;22:333.
52. Cadiere GB, Rajan A, Rqibate M, et al. Endoluminal fundoplication (ELF)—evolution of EsophyX, a new surgical device for transoral surgery. Minim Invasive Ther Allied Technol 2006;15:348.
53. Cadiere GB, Van Sante N, Graves JE, et al. Two-year results of a feasibility study on antireflux transoral incisionless fundoplication using EsophyX. Surg Endosc 2009;23:957.
54. Bergman S, Mikami DJ, Hazey JW, et al. Endolumenal fundoplication with EsophyX: the initial North American experience. Surg Innov 2008;15:166.
55. Ramage JI, Rothstein RI, Edmundowicz SA, et al. Endoscopically placed titanium plicator for GERD: pivotal phase—preliminary 6-month results [abstract]. Gastrointest Endosc 2006;63:126.

56. Sud R, Puri R, Chung S, et al. The His-Wiz antireflux procedure results in symptomatic and pH improvement at 1 year of follow-up [abstract]. Gastrointest Endosc 2006;63:13.
57. Kauer WK, Roy-Shapira A, Watson D, et al. Preclinical trial of a modified gastroscope that performs a true anterior fundoplication for the endoluminal treatment of gastroesophageal reflux disease. Surg Endosc 2009 [Epub ahead of print].

Recent Advances in the Use of Stents for Esophageal Disease

Drew B. Schembre, MD, FASGE, FACG[a,b,*]

KEYWORDS

- Esophageal stent • Dysphagia • Esophageal cancer
- Esophageal stricture • Esophageal perforation
- Esophageal fistula

Esophageal cancer causes a unique type of misery. Beyond all the other disabilities and anxieties that come with a cancer diagnosis, patients with malignant dysphagia often feel like they are starving to death. Patients often report avoiding eating even though hungry, because of pain or choking sensations, and may present for treatment only after significant weight loss. Undernutrition itself is one of the strongest predictors of survival in patients with esophageal cancer anticipating treatment.[1] To make matters worse, esophageal cancer patients may suffer embarrassment and isolation when they cannot participate in the many social and family activities revolving around meals. Individuals with tight, benign strictures also share some of these handicaps. Although not facing the same grave prognosis, these individuals also experience weight loss, aspiration, and pain as well as frustration, anxiety, and decreased quality of life, especially if they have to undergo frequent endoscopic dilation.

Given the level of desperation caused by dysphagia, combined with the easy access of the esophagus, esophageal dilation was probably one of the earliest successful gastrointestinal interventions. It is easy to imagine some unfortunate prehistoric human using a stick or bone to dislodge a piece of meat in the first esophageal dilation. Through much of recorded history, wax candles and other tapered, rigid devices have been used for the same purpose. Because dilation alone provides only temporary relief in most cases of malignant dysphagia, early prostheses or stents were constructed out of smooth, rigid materials such as ivory, sandalwood,

The author has no conflicts to report in the preparation of this article. The author has received speaking honoraria from Olympus America, Fujinon, Cook Endoscopy, and Boston Scientific, Inc.

a Division of Gastroenterology, Virginia Mason Medical Center, 1100 9th Avenue, MS:C3, Seattle, WA 98101, USA
b University of Washington, Seattle, WA, USA
* Corresponding author. Division of Gastroenterology, Virginia Mason Medical Center, 1100 9th Avenue, MS:C3, Seattle, WA 98101, USA.
E-mail address: drew.schembre@vmmc.org

and bone. Esophageal stents evolved slowly over the first part of the twentieth century, with the use of rubber and plastics. Innovation has exploded over the last 20 years with the development of the self-expanding metal stent (SEMS). Constructed from surgical steel or, more commonly, a shape-retaining nickel and titanium alloy, nitinol, SEMS are easy to place and have quickly replaced rigid stents in the treatment of esophageal malignancies. Further modifications in stent materials, such as the construction of self-expanding plastic stents (SEPS) and even biodegradable materials, have spawned a rapid increase in the use of removable stents for benign conditions such as refractory strictures, perforations, and fistulas (**Fig. 1**).

This article describes the current experience with esophageal stenting for malignant and benign conditions, and examines new innovations in stent design and applications.

STENTS FOR MALIGNANCY

The primary application for esophageal stents remains the treatment of malignant dysphagia. While the incidence of new esophageal cancers has remained relatively stable over the past 10 years at about 4.5 new cases per 100,000 people, adenocarcinoma has rapidly replaced squamous cell cancer as the primary malignancy.[2,3] Squamous cell cancers remain a major source of mortality worldwide, with over 400,000 new cases each year, mostly in developing countries. Esophageal cancers internationally rank as the fourth most common cause of cancer mortality among men and the seventh most common cause among women.[4] Adenocarcinoma arising from Barrett's esophagus tends to develop more distally, but otherwise the complaints and complications associated with the 2 malignancies are similar. Most patients present with dysphagia and weight loss as their main complaints. Because tumor usually occupies over half of the esophageal lumen when dysphagia develops, most these cancers will be unresectable at the time of diagnosis. Treatment, therefore, often focuses on palliation of symptoms as well as attempts at improving nutrition, in the hope of at least marginally improving survival. Although esophagectomy may be performed to relieve dysphagia, undertaking a large operation in the setting of metastatic disease is discouraged because of associated morbidity and mortality, as well as a reduction in quality of life, without extending survival.[5,6] Even after esophagectomy for localized esophageal cancer, many patients will experience recurrence locally or at distant sites, with 5-year survival hovering around 20%.[7] Benign strictures of the esophagogastric anastomosis occur in at least 20% of those who undergo

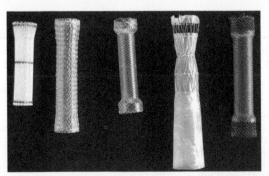

Fig. 1. A variety of partially and fully covered metal and plastic stents. From left Polyflex, Alimaxx, Niti-S, Dua Antireflux, Evolution.

surgery, although these rarely require stenting.[8] Chemotherapy and radiation therapy can often effectively improve swallowing in many patients; however, many of these patients will suffer from recurrent esophageal obstruction if tumor recurs locally. A portion of those who undergo esophagectomy for cure also experience local recurrence and require palliation. Several other cancers can cause dysphagia, including primary lung cancer, proximal gastric cancer, and a variety of cancers that metastasize to mediastinal lymph nodes.[9] Feeding tubes may be inserted below the obstruction to maintain adequate caloric intake; however, risks of aspiration persist and most people, even those with terminal diseases, simply want to eat.

RIGID STENTS

A discussion of new developments in esophageal stents merits a brief mention of older-style rigid stents. Although SEMS largely replaced rigid stents in the 1990s, in many developing countries rigid stents are still widely used. The low cost of rigid stents stands as the only real advantage of these devices. Commercially available rigid stents generally sell for as little as a few dollars, or can be fashioned out of rubber or polyethylene tubing for pennies. However, the cost of the stent is offset by numerous disadvantages. Rigid stents require stricture dilation up to 18 mm before placement, and heavy sedation is frequently necessary before driving them into position. Not surprisingly, perforations are common, with reported rates of 8% or higher.[10] Despite their generous exterior diameter, most rigid stents provide an internal lumen of only 12 mm or less, as several millimeters of wall thickness are needed to prevent collapse. Rigid plastic stents also seem to lead to more frequent interventions such as disimpaction of food, bleeding, and migration than SEMS, ultimately leading to higher cumulative costs.[11,12] Although rigid stents are technically removable, this is rarely performed.

SELF-EXPANDABLE METAL STENTS

The appeal of stenting with SEMS lies in their relative simplicity; as the stent expands, it pushes the tumor aside and allows food to pass almost immediately. The truth, of course, is that stenting with SEMS can be a complex undertaking with risks, discomfort, and limitations of effectiveness. Early enthusiasm for SEMS as a panacea for malignant dysphagia waned somewhat as reports of complications, stent migration, and reocclusion surfaced. Despite many modifications and overall stent evolution over the last 20 years, complication rates have not changed dramatically.[13]

Nonetheless stents remain tremendously appealing, in part because of limitations of other therapies. Unfortunately, only a few studies have looked at the relative effectiveness of different therapies for malignant dysphagia. There is broad recognition that endoscopic dilation of malignant strictures can alleviate dysphagia only for short periods. Complication rates—primarily for perforations—increase with larger, more sclerotic strictures, more aggressive dilation, and after radiotherapy.[14] There does not seem to be a difference in efficacy or complication rates between dilation with wire-guided Savary-type dilators or balloon devices.[15] Chemotherapy combined with radiation can improve survival in patients with both early and advanced-stage esophageal cancer, and can be very effective for controlling malignant dysphagia. In one large study, dysphagia resolved in 77% of patients with Stage III or IV disease after 5-fluorouracil, mitomycin C, and external beam radiation, and persisted until death in 60%. Median dysphagia-free duration was 5 months.[16] Single-dose brachytherapy seems to provide equal or better initial relief of malignant dysphagia than stent placement,[17] except in patients with particularly advanced disease, multiple comorbidities, and short life expectancy.[18]

An abstract by Canto and colleagues[19] suggested that treatment of malignant dysphagia with SEMS cost about a third of treatment with photodynamic therapy, and a trial of thermal ablation using Nd:YAG laser or argon plasma coagulation versus SEMS suggested lower cost but reduced quality of life in the SEMS group.[20]

In general, the use of permanent stents should be reserved for patients with dysphagia secondary to advanced malignancy who are either not candidates for, or unwilling to undergo, surgery, chemotherapy, or radiotherapy, or who have experienced a recurrence after definitive treatment. Stents should extend about 2 cm proximal and distal to the tumor. Fortunately, most stents are sold in a variety of lengths to accommodate a broad spectrum of tumors. Partially covered stents have largely replaced uncovered stents for most indications, as they have been shown to delay tumor ingrowth longer without greater risk of migration. The main contraindication for esophageal stent placement is poor performance status, with life expectancy of less than 4 weeks. Relative contraindications include tumors within 2 cm of the upper esophageal sphincter, uncorrectable coagulopathy, or tumor invasion of the aorta or airways. Previous stent migration is not a contraindication, but does signal a need to try a larger or different type of stent or to use a securing device. Placement of standard stents within 2 cm of the upper esophageal sphincter has been associated with airway compromise, persistent discomfort, and osteomyelitis of the cervical vertebrae from pressure necrosis.[21,22] Smaller-diameter stents custom designed for the cervical esophagus are available in some countries, and stents sold for use in the upper airway or bile ducts have been used successfully in the hypopharynx (Fig. 2).[23] The caveat for placing these stents is that without flared ends, they are more likely to migrate, and the exposed tines of biliary stents may cause pain and irritation. Many experts now suggest that standard esophageal stents can also be used close to the upper esophageal sphincter, as long as these patients are followed closely and recognize the risk of complications.[24]

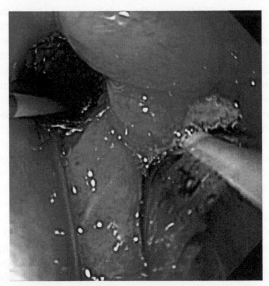

Fig. 2. Covered biliary stent deployed at the hypopharynx. Endotrachial tube seen in place at the level of the vocal cords.

Stenting across the lower esophageal sphincter poses its own challenges. Stents in this position may be more likely to migrate and can lead to free reflux of stomach contents. Attempts to incorporate antireflux mechanisms into SEMS have met with mixed reviews. The addition of a "windsock" to the distal end of a SEMS was intended to reduce free reflux from the stomach when a stent is placed across the esophago-gastric junction by inverting and creating a partial barrier. Antegrade passage of food and liquids is generally unencumbered, and an inverted windsock can usually be straightened with a gulp of water.[25] The windsock and other variations of an antireflux stent probably do reduce exposure of the proximal esophagus and airways to regurgitated gastric and duodenal contents compared with standard stents[26]; however, no overall improvement in survival or reduction in severe complications has been demonstrated.[27]

Physicians have historically avoided placing stents in patients who anticipate chemo- or radiotherapy, as tumor response to treatment may lead to stent migration. In addition, scatter from metal stents may complicate radiation dosimetry. Further, pressure from an in-dwelling stent may increase the risk of fistula formation during chemo- or radiotherapy.[28] More recently, studies have shown that removable stents can be used during neoadjuvant chemo-radiotherapy to help patients avoid nutritional compromise as well as the need for a jejunal feeding tube during the several weeks of treatment leading up to esophagectomy.[29] In a recent series, Siddiqui and colleagues[30] retrospectively compared 12 patients who underwent placement of SEPS in 24 patients who had J-tube placement before neoadjuvant therapy and esophagectomy for locally advanced esophageal cancer. No difference was seen in complication rates, weight gain, or the ability to undergo successful surgery between the 2 groups; however all but one of the patients who had SEPS were able to resume oral alimentation.

SELF-EXPANDABLE METAL STENTS FOR MALIGNANT DISEASE

Placing SEMS has become standard therapy for palliation of malignant dysphagia. However, despite the seeming simplicity of placing an expandable tube in a luminal restriction, the complexity of tumor behavior and esophageal physiology has forced numerous stent design modifications. Original SEMS, such as the Esophacoil, produced a high level of radial force. Persistent discomfort was common, and reports emerged of pressure necrosis and fistula formation. SEMS woven from high-memory alloys such as nitinol allowed for production of a softer stent, which nonetheless opened the lumen with slow, constant radial force. Unfortunately, the tumor often grew through the open mesh and dysphagia recurred, sometimes within a few weeks. To combat this problem, stents were wrapped with a silicone or plastic cover. The ends of the stent were left uncovered to allow healthy mucosa to overgrow the exposed wire in order to prevent late migration. Migration within the first few days remained a problem, and designs were further modified to incorporate proximal and distal flares or "dog bone" shapes to combat this. Covered SEMS have virtually replaced uncovered stents for almost all esophageal applications. Covered stents also emerged as an excellent treatment for malignant fistulas, and have become the standard of care for treatment of malignant esophagobronchial leaks, sometimes with a second stent placed in the airway.[13] The ability to use partially covered stents to treat benign fistulas and perforations had been limited by difficulty in removing the devices once tissue has overgrown the open portion of the stent. Protruding wire ends of the original SEMS helped reduce migration; however, their tendency to project laterally into the esophageal wall immediately after deployment compromised the ability to safely reposition or remove the stent if it were misdeployed. Rounded, continuous struts at the ends of stents allow them to move with traction via grasping forceps immediately after deployment. The incorporation of a purse-string suture at the proximal end of the stent is a welcome innovation. By pulling on the suture with forceps, the proximal end of the stent collapses, allowing the endoscopist to pull the entire stent higher in the esophagus or remove it completely. Displacing the stent distally can be more difficult, but can usually be accomplished by grasping distal tines with forceps, or inflating a dilating balloon within the stent and applying gentle pressure. However, once epithelium has grown over the uncovered portion of the stent, repositioning or removal becomes much more difficult. In fact, excessive growth of benign epithelium at the ends of SEMS remains the most common cause of recurrent dysphagia, with hypertrophic mucosa leading to at least partial occlusion of the lumen in up to one-half of patients at 2 months.[31] Fully covered metal stents and SEPS were designed in part to address this problem but also to facilitate repositioning and even late removal, thus opening up a broad array of new, benign applications. With these stents, occlusion by benign tissue overgrowth does seem to occur less frequently, or at least later, but at the cost of more frequent migration. In a recent study comparing partially covered metal stents to fully covered metal and plastic stents, SEPS migrated in 29% of patients compared with 17% for the partially covered Ultraflex stent and 12% for the double-layer Niti-S stent.[31] Further modifications have been made to the outer surface of some fully covered stents in an attempt to increase adhesion and decrease migration. The Alimaxx fully covered metal stent incorporates many small "herringbone" flanges on the outer surface of the stent, and the Tai-Woo double stent features a fully coated metal inner stent surrounded by an uncovered outer metal stent. Several new fully covered metal stents have either recently been introduced or will become available soon. The relative merits of differences in design will need to be studied. Further, the benefit of any of the fully covered stents over partially covered stents for malignant disease remains to be determined.

Many endoscopists use endoscopically placed clips at the proximal margin of newly placed stents over the exposed wire, or directly clipping the purse-string suture to the esophageal mucosa, to reduce the chance of early migration. Reliable data on the effectiveness of this technique is lacking; however, it is a relatively simple and safe intervention, and may help the endoscopist rest easier.

COMPLICATIONS

In addition to stent migration and benign tissue overgrowth, other complications have been associated with esophageal stents. Kozarek and colleagues[32] described the propensity for the development of late problems from SEMS in 1992, and numerous other articles since then have documented a broad array of potential complications including chest pain, perforation, fistula development, intestinal obstruction after migration, hemorrhage, epidural abscess, aspiration, and stent fracture.[33–35] Debate continues over the relative risks of complications after stenting in patients who have undergone prior chemo- or radiotherapy; however, because there are few good palliative options for these individuals, stenting remains the mainstay of treatment.[36,37]

STENTS FOR BENIGN DISEASE

As described earlier, uncovered and partially covered stents have not played a signif-icant role in benign esophageal diseases because of their tendency to rapidly embed themselves in the esophageal wall, making removal difficult and dangerous. Left long term, these stents may erode, occlude, fistulize, or cause other severe problems. However, with the introduction of a fully coated, removable plastic stent (Polyflex, Boston Scientific), a host of new applications has been attempted, with varying success. Fully coated metal stents have followed, and although they do not generally carry formal indications for temporary stenting in benign diseases, many of these devices have been placed to treat benign conditions with the expectation of eventual stent removal.

STRICTURES

Although most peptic inflammatory esophageal strictures respond to simple dilation, a subset of benign strictures recurs or even worsens despite aggressive treatment. These injuries may include strictures from caustic injury, radiation, complications from esophageal surgery or endoscopic therapies such as mucosal resection, submucosal dissection, or photodynamic therapy. Therapies have included repeated endoscopic or self-bougenage, dilation combined with steroid injection, hyperbaric therapy, or radial incision followed by dilation, with variable rates of sustained improvement. Because stents can successfully treat malignant strictures, the idea of using stents for benign disease has appeal. In theory, an expandable stent within a recalcitrant benign stricture would have an advantage over simple dilation by allowing the disrupted fibrous tissue to remodel over the fixed platform of the stent, rather than simply tearing scar tissue and allowing it to heal unsupported. Until recently, removing the stent once healing had occurred has been the major stumbling block. Nevertheless, some experts still advocate use of partially covered SEMS for up to 16 weeks for treating very proximal and distal strictures where migration with fully covered SEPS is more common.[24,38–41] Endoscopic inspection of these stents is suggested at 4-week intervals to detect the beginnings of tissue overgrowth of the open mesh, and to remove the stent—and place a new SEMS—if this occurs. Despite some limited enthusiasm for SEMS, SEPS have largely replaced partially covered SEMS for treating recalcitrant esophageal strictures. The Polyflex stent is constructed of polyester mesh completely covered with a silicone membrane, and has a flaring proximal end to reduce migration. Because the stent is fully covered, tissue ingrowth does not occur. Further, the use of plastic and silicone probably provokes less of a granulation reaction than metal, further reducing the amount of tissue buildup at the margins of the stent.[42] The Polyflex stent deforms into an ellipse with traction, decreasing the diameter of the proximal flared end, which enables removal by pulling slowly and continuously with grasping forceps. The inner surface is smooth, whereas a textured outer surface may help decrease migration. Three radiopaque bands facilitate visualization during deployment.

Placing a SEPS into a benign stricture can be somewhat more challenging than placing a SEMS. First, the SEPS must be loaded on the delivery system by pulling it into a plastic sleeve with a netlike grasping catheter. Care must be taken at this step to ensure the stent loads smoothly and does not fold on itself, as this can compromise uniform expansion on deployment. The delivery system is also stiffer and has a wider diameter than most SEMS, necessitating prior dilation of the stricture to at least 12 mm before placement. SEPS are less visible fluoroscopically, and have tendency to shorten and squirt out of the delivery catheter at the end of deployment as the device rapidly expands. This action may propel the stent beyond the stricture. It is important to carefully watch the position of the stent as it passes from the delivery device, often maintaining traction on the partially deployed stent. However, if the stent does misdeploy distally, it can often be repositioned endoscopically with grasping forceps and traction. Repositioning a proximally displaced SEPS is more difficult, and it is usually better to simply remove the stent, wash it off, reload it into the delivery system, and try again. SEPS have greater radial force than SEMS but still may require several hours to fully expand. Care should be taken when removing the tapered tip of the delivery device, as this can dislodge the stent proximally. Advancing the delivery sheath distally to the proximal edge of the deployed stent to brace it as the tip is withdrawn through the narrowed portion of the stent may help prevent displacement.

Most series have reported high rates of technical success for SEPS delivery, and immediate improvement in dysphagia. In an early series, Radecke and colleagues[43] reported technical success in placing 50 SEPS in 39 patients with a variety of malignant and benign stenoses and fistulas, with 4 initial failures due to patient intolerance or maldeployment. Ultimately, 69% of these patients were able to resume eating while an additional 15% could handle their secretions but could not eat. Another 15% of placements were deemed unsuccessful. Many small, retrospective series have reported high levels of initial technical success, but long-term relief of dysphagia has been highly variable. Evrard and colleagues[44] reported that 17 of 21 patients (81%) achieved substantial improvement at 21 months after stent removal for a variety of benign strictures. Repici and colleagues[45] similarly noted that 12 of 15 (80%) patients with benign strictures in whom SEPS were placed were able to go without additional dilation for the almost 2 years after stent removal. However, most other series have reported lower long-term success. Holm and colleagues[46] reported only 17% durable response among 30 patients who had a variety of anastomotic, postradiation, and other strictures (including 9 with fistulas) after a total of 83 stents were placed. At the author's institution, reasonable relief of dysphagia was achieved among an initial group of 11 patients with a difficult collection of benign strictures after placement of 16 SEPS for an average of 52 days.[47] After removal of SEPS, 6 (55%) patients (2 with recalcitrant reflux strictures and 2 with stenotic anastomoses) required no further dilation. One patient with a radiation-induced stricture developed a fistula that required permanent stenting, and another required continued periodic dilation after stent removal. In another larger, retrospective series, 64 patients with benign anastomotic, radiation, or peptic strictures were treated with SEPS. Lasting success was achieved in only 17% of patients.[46] Although no severe complications were reported, SEPS migrated from 82% of peptic strictures and 75% of anastomotic strictures, but only 25% of radiation-induced strictures. Migration was more common among distal and proximal strictures compared with mid-esophageal locations.

In the only prospective trial of SEPS, Dua and colleagues[48] reported a modest 32% lasting improvement of dysphagia after stent removal among 40 patients with anastomotic, caustic, radiation, and other types of benign strictures after an average 4-week insertion. These patients had undergone a mean of 12 dilations each before stent placement. Stent placement was unsuccessful in 2 patients and complications were common, with 22% migration, 8% bleeding, 11% severe chest pain, 3% fistula, and 6% in whom the stent could not be safely removed. In reported series of SEPS for benign diseases, stent migration remains the most common complication, occurring in over half of the cases.[40,41,49] Although this problem can usually be treated easily, and at times results from a successful dilation of a stricture, it invariably requires repeat endoscopy, often with dilation, extraction, and placement of another stent. A variety of techniques has been attempted to reduce migration, including clipping the stent itself or sutures tied through the stent to the esophageal wall (**Fig. 3**).[50] In the author's experience, this may reduce the frequency of initial migration; however, the durability of traditional endoclipping to mucosa is limited, especially if a thick piece of covered stent is contained in the clip. These pieces tend to detach within a few hours to days, and

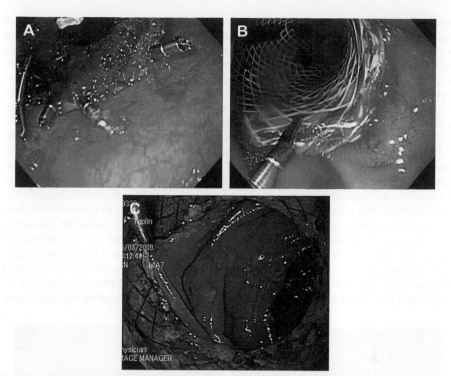

Fig. 3. (A) Multiple endoclips at the proximal margin of a Niti-S stent. (B) Single clip on a Polyflex stent. (C) Single clip at the distal end of a fully covered stent.

probably do not reduce the incidence of stent migration appreciably. Reports have surfaced of ways to modify these stents by cutting holes in the lining or sewing sutures into the proximal end to enhance the security of clips, although the overall effectiveness of these techniques remains uncertain.[51] One group of creative endoscopists tied a long suture to the proximal end of a fully covered stent, then after deployment passed it out of the patient's mouth and tied it around his ear.[52] Although possibly effective, it is doubtful that this technique will attract a wide following.

Other complications associated with SEPS have been more serious, including perforations, bleeding, fistulas, and an inability to remove stents.[53] These complications may be related to the relatively large diameter and stiffness of the insertion device. SEPS themselves produce more radial force than SEMS and may cause more discomfort as a result. This situation occasionally necessitates premature stent removal, although most patients can be controlled with oral pain medication.

An attempt to counter the shortcomings of SEPS inevitably led to the development of fully covered metal stents, or what has awkwardly been termed FCSEMS. Experience with these hybrid stents is limited. A recent report by Eloubeidi and Lopes[54] detailed 7 patients with refractory, benign esophageal strictures who underwent temporary stenting with an Alimaxx stent, an internally fully covered metal device. Stent placement and removal was successful in all patients; however, only 2 (29%) patients showed sustained improvement in dysphagia. Stent migration in the larger series of 31 patients with a mix of benign and malignant conditions occurred in 36% of patients. Migration was more common if the stent crossed the EG junction (59% vs 16%). Conio and colleagues[23] have reported using custom-made, 10- to 14-mm proximal flaring Niti-S

SEMS in either a fully covered or partially covered design for postradiation strictures of the hypopharynx. In this series, 6 of 7 patients experienced immediate and persistent improvement in profound dysphagia after placement of a modified Niti-S stent. These stents were well tolerated, easily removed, and led to lasting improvement in dysphagia at an average of 4 months after removal without additional intervention. One patient developed an esophagotracheal fistula that required permanent stenting, and 5 stents migrated at a median of 3 months. The author has used covered biliary SEMS with a diameter of 8 to 10 mm for the same indication, with good initial results in 5 cases of complete occlusion of the proximal esophagus (**Fig. 4**).[55] The author graduated to a 12- or 16-mm bronchial Polyflex stent in 2 cases. One patient developed cervical osteomyelitis requiring early stent removal and subsequent restenosis, and another developed an anterior neck abscess that resolved with simple drainage. Four of the 5 were able to maintain oral alimentation, albeit with periodic self- or endoscopic dilation. Tai-Woo has recently entered the United States market with a removable, fully covered Niti-S metal stent in a variety of lengths and diameters; however, published results are still forthcoming. In initial experience with this device in 10 patients, the author found it easy to deploy and remove from within benign strictures and fistulas. Stents migrated in 40% of patients, but no other serious complications occurred (**Fig. 5**). Among 2 patients with recalcitrant benign strictures, 1 has remained free of dysphagia after stent removal.[56] Fully covered metal stents from other manufacturers

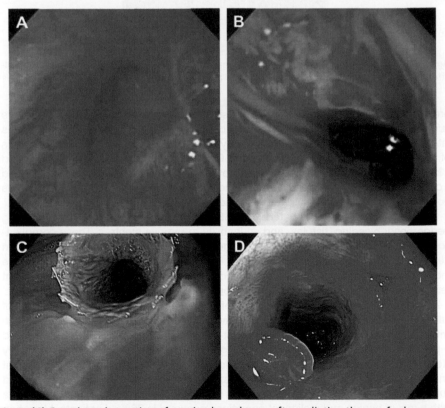

Fig. 4. (*A*) Complete obstruction of proximal esophagus after radiation therapy for laryngeal cancer. (*B*) Post dilation after blind puncture with an endoscopic ultrasound needle. (*C*) Covered biliary stent in place. (*D*) Post stent removal.

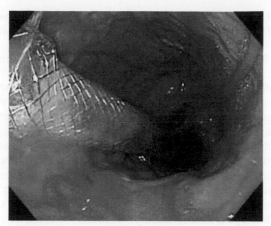

Fig. 5. Migrated Niti-S stent.

are expected in the near future. Ultimately, success with benign strictures probably has more to do with the degree of underlying tissue damage than any particular type of stent. Longer, denser, and more fibrotic strictures will probably recur after even prolonged stent dilation.

FISTULAS AND PERFORATIONS

Although results from the stenting of benign strictures have been disappointing, temporary stenting for perforations and fistulas has shown very favorable results. Palliative permanent metal stenting for malignant fistulas and perforations has been standard of care for the last 10 years, and numerous series have demonstrated the effectiveness of this strategy.[13] Because of these successes, stent placement for benign esophageal leaks has become more common. At present, placement of a potentially removable stent has become the first-line treatment for perforations and fistulas in many centers in the United States. This sea change has come in part due to the mortality associated with untreated perforations, which has been estimated at 20% to 45%.[57] Although aggressive surgical treatment may double or triple survival, some patients may not be ideal surgical candidates due to delayed diagnosis, age, recent anastomoses, and so forth.[58,59] Primary endoscopic repair of perforations of the esophagus using endoclips, tissue glues, and endoscopic suturing devices have been reported[60]; however, these techniques are usually reserved for acute perforations or fistulas limited to a few millimeters. Larger and more chronic defects usually require diversion, either surgically or by placement of an occlusive stent combined with mediastinal debridement and drainage. Virtually all currently available partially covered metal stents have been used to seal perforations and fistulas, and many have been successfully removed in the setting of benign diseases.[61–64] Just as with the treatment of benign strictures, problems arise when removing these stents, as tissue growth through the uncovered portion of the stent can adhere the stent to the esophageal wall. Complications such as bleeding,[65] fistula formation,[66] and even segmental amputation of the esophageal wall[67] have been reported with attempts at removing partially covered stents. Some SEMS may be easier to remove than others. Ultraflex stents can often be grasped distally and invaginated,[60] and Z-stents may be wedged free by grasping the proximal edge and advancing an overtube around it.[68] It has also been reported that SEMS with extensive granulation tissue overgrowth can be removed after placement of a second

SEPS within the SEMS, and waiting 2 to 3 weeks for the pressure of the internal SEPS to cause necrosis of the granulation tissue and allow simple withdrawal of both stents together.[69]

Introduction of SEPS has clearly increased the willingness of endoscopists to treat esophageal leaks. Placement is usually straightforward, and the stent can be removed easily once the defect has closed, or sooner if it is unsuccessful or complications arise. Several small series have documented the success of SEPS for this indication. In Germany Hünerbein and colleagues[70] reported an early series of 9 patients who developed leaks after esophagectomy. Stents were left in place for an average of 29 days and began oral intake around day 11. There was no mortality (compared with 20% mortality in a similar group treated conservatively without stenting), and at 12-month follow-up no structuring or leaks had occurred. Freeman and colleagues[71] described 17 patients who suffered iatrogenic perforations of the esophagus (8 during endoscopy and 9 from surgery) over 2 years, who underwent immediate stenting with a SEPS combined with mediastinal drainage where necessary. Initial sealing of the leak was achieved in 16 patients (94%) by esophagram, and 14 (82%) were able to initiate oral nutrition within 72 hours. Four stents required replacement or repositioning after migration, and all stents were removed at an average of 52 days with leak closure in all but 1 patient who was treated surgically. In the author's institution, 6 of 6 benign leaks resolved completely after SEPS placement for an average of 5 weeks.[47] Leaks do best with any therapy when they are treated immediately. Spontaneous esophageal perforation (Boerhaave syndrome) and other leaks associated with extensive soilage do less well but have shown reasonable rates of healing after placement of SEPS. An early case report of SEPS for a patient with delayed presentation of Boerhaave syndrome showed that this nonsurgical intervention could be effective even in the setting of extensive mediastinal involvement, as long as adequate drainage was provided.[72] A series of 32 patients with a mix of postsurgical and spontaneous perforations, over half of whom failed initial attempts at surgical closure, underwent treatment with SEPS, resulting in functional sealing of 78% of patients and successful closure in 70%.[73]

Limited experience has been generated with fully covered SEMS for treating esophageal leaks. Alimaxx stents were used to treat 8 patients with tracheoesophageal fistulas, with a 63% success rate. Two of 2 postoperative leaks treated with this device sealed completely, whereas only 1 of 2 perforations treated with the Alimaxx stent healed.[54] The author has successfully used the Alimaxx stent to treat leaks, but has occasionally found them difficult to remove after several weeks, with stents breaking apart and having to be removed piecemeal (**Fig. 6**). Fully covered Niti-S stents have also been used successfully for this indication, with 4 of 5 anastomotic and other benign fistulas remaining closed after stent removal.[56]

SEPS and fully covered SEMS are being placed in more severe disruptions. Amrani and colleagues[74] reported the use of SEPS to close a variety of large esophageal and colonic disruptions, some approaching complete disunion of the organ. The author has had similar success with patients with near complete separation of gastroesophageal anastomoses following bariatric and other types of surgery (**Fig. 7**). As long as the seal is complete and the surrounding area remains well drained complete healing may be the rule. Further studies will be necessary to define what stents are best for which problems, how to maximize the initial seal and, perhaps more important, how to reduce migration among fully covered stents.

Stenting for benign diseases has evolved from the difficult removal of permanent stents to easier removal of temporary stents (albeit with a tradeoff of higher migration rates) to, more recently, the development of biodegradable stents that require no removal at all. Although the idea of biodegradable stents has been around for over

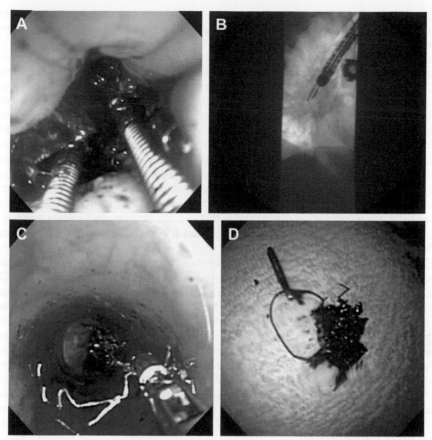

Fig. 6. (A) Removal of an Alimaxx stent with 2 grasping forceps. (B) Fluoroscopic view. (C) Fractured stent. (D) Stent fragment with endoclip still in place on purse-string suture.

10 years, newer designs and materials may finally allow more widespread use of the devices. Small series from Japan and Europe have shown utility of biodegradable stents. Saito and colleagues[75] used an "ultraflex-type" stent made of knitted poly-L-lactic acid monofilaments in 13 patients for a variety of indications. Six stenoses

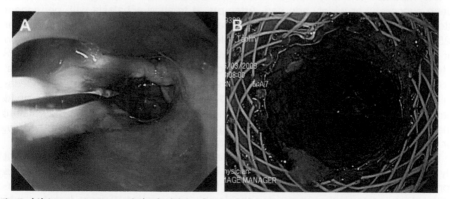

Fig. 7. (A) Large anastomotic leak. (B) Leak covered with Polyflex overlapping a Niti-S stent.

(2 caustic, 4 anastomotic) and 7 large-area mucosectomy had biodegradable stents placed without difficulty. Stents dissolved and migrated in most cases between 2 and 3 weeks; however, none of these patients developed a primary stricture or restenosis at up to 2 years of follow-up. Whereas it can be argued that the strictures treated may have responded to other measures, the idea of a prophylactic, dissolving stent after mucosectomy is intriguing. To date, the greatest obstacle to large-area mucosectomy in the esophagus, whether by endoscopic mucosal resection or endoscopic submucosal dissection, has been the high rate of stenosis once an area greater than about two-thirds the circumference of the esophagus has been removed, with stenosis occurring in 70% to 80% of patients in whom complete circumferential resection has taken place.[76] If a scaffold could be created that would reliably prevent stenosis, more aggressive resections would likely follow. Investigators have successfully used removable SEPS coated with an animal urinary bladder extracellular matrix (ECM) to encourage neoepithelialization without stenosis in animal models. More recently, these investigators dispensed with the stent entirely, and simply wrapped a glue-coated ECM around an inflatable balloon and deployed it over the mucosal defect, with good success.[77]

Other case reports and abstracts have described the use of biodegradable stents.[75,78] An English group reported the use of a polydioxanone stent (Ella-BD, ELLA-CS, Hradec Karlove, Czech Republic) in 4 patients with refractory benign esophageal strictures.[79] Despite some difficulty with deployment of early designs, all patients were dysphagia-free at short follow-up after insertion (4–17 weeks). In a larger series using the same type of stent, Repici and colleagues[80] described placing the Ella-BD stent in 12 patients with refractory benign strictures. Stents were successfully placed in all patients, with one episode of minor bleeding and a 17% early migration rate. Stents were still visible in half of the patients at 3 months. No long-term results were available; however, 2 of 12 patients had recurrent dysphagia at median follow-up of 22 weeks. These are clearly very early studies, and more information will need to be gathered concerning this type and other types of biodegradable esophageal stents.

Although drug-eluting stents are popular for endovascular applications, the concept has been slow to catch on for esophageal stenting. One recent animal study demonstrated that SEMS coated with the antiproliferative chemotherapy agent paclitaxel provoked very little local tissue reaction after 4 weeks in the esophagi of 7 dogs, and were easily separated from the esophageal tissue and removed.[81] No human trials have been reported, but are likely forthcoming.

It is important to briefly mention stent applications in the esophagus that have not been successful or widely adopted. Attempts at treating achalasia with permanent stents were unsuccessful due to high rates of complications.[82] A large-diameter (25 mm) fully covered SEMS with a deflatable balloon at the distal end for localization at the cardia was used to treat 15 patients with poorly controlled variceal bleeding.[83] Stents were left in place for 2 to 14 days, and removed after management of patients' portal hypertension was otherwise "optimized." Ultimately, all stents were successfully removed without complication, rebleeding, or mortality. Although this seems to have been a successful study, it remains unclear whether this would be more useful than other forms of endotherapy for bleeding varices, such as banding, sclerotherapy, or even temporary placement of a traction-type tamponade balloon.

In summary, while expandable stents remain highly useful for palliation of malignant dysphasia, evolution of stent materials and design have broadened the applications for the devices to encompass a host of benign conditions. Treatment of benign esophageal strictures and leaks has grown considerably over the last 10 years, largely due to the creation of easily removable stents. Removable stents are also being used in malignant disease as a bridge to surgery or other therapies. Complication rates for malignant and benign applications remain significant, and careful patient selection and close monitoring are essential. New designs may help reduce these complication rates. Additional advances may enable stent placement as prophylaxis for large-area mucosal resection and dissection procedures. Newer applications will no doubt arise as technology improves.

REFERENCES

1. Lecleire S, Di Fiore F, Antonietti M, et al. Undernutrition is predictive of early mortality after palliative self-expanding metal stent insertion in patients with inoperable or recurrent esophageal cancer. Gastrointest Endosc 2006;64(4): 479–84.
2. Surveillance Epidemiology and End Results. Available at: http://seer.cancer.gov. Accessed June, 2009.
3. Jemal A, Thomas A, Murray T, et al. Cancer statistics, 2002. CA Cancer J Clin 2002;52(1):23–47.
4. Parkin DM, Bray F, Ferlay J, et al. Global cancer statistics, 2002. CA Cancer J Clin 2005;55(2):74–108.
5. Birkmeyer JD, Siewers AE, Finlayson EV, et al. Hospital volume and surgical mortality in the United States. N Engl J Med 2002;346(15):1128–37.
6. Baba M, Aikou T, Natsugoe S, et al. Appraisal of ten-year survival following esophagectomy for carcinoma of the esophagus with emphasis on quality of life. World J Surg 1997;21(3):282–5 [discussion: 86].
7. Urba SG, Orringer MB, Turrisi A, et al. Randomized trial of preoperative chemo-radiation versus surgery alone in patients with locoregional esophageal carcinoma. J Clin Oncol 2001;19(2):305–13.
8. Collins G, Johnson E, Kroshus T, et al. Experience with minimally invasive esophagectomy. Surg Endosc 2006;20(2):298–301.
9. Sanchez AA, Wu TT, Prieto VG, et al. Comparison of primary and metastatic malignant melanoma of the esophagus: clinicopathologic review of 10 cases. Arch Pathol Lab Med 2008;132(10):1623–9.
10. Tytgat GN, Tytgat S. Esophageal endoprosthesis in malignant stricture. J Gastroenterol 1994;29(Suppl 7):80–4.
11. Davies N, Thomas HG, Eyre-Brook IA. Palliation of dysphagia from inoperable oesophageal carcinoma using Atkinson tubes or self-expanding metal stents. Ann R Coll Surg Engl 1998;80(6):394–7.
12. O'Donnell CA, Fullarton GM, Watt E, et al. Randomized clinical trial comparing self-expanding metallic stents with plastic endoprostheses in the palliation of oesophageal cancer. Br J Surg 2002;89(8):985–92.
13. Ross WA, Alkassab F, Lynch PM, et al. Evolving role of self-expanding metal stents in the treatment of malignant dysphagia and fistulas. Gastrointest Endosc 2007;65(1):70–6.
14. Schembre DB, Kozarek RA. Endoscopic therapeutic esophageal interventions. Curr Opin Gastroenterol 2000;16(4):380–5.
15. Reed CE. Pitfalls and complications of esophageal prosthesis, laser therapy, and dilation. Chest Surg Clin N Am 1997;7(3):623–36.
16. Coia LR, Engstrom PF, Paul AR, et al. Long-term results of infusional 5-FU, mitomycin-C and radiation as primary management of esophageal carcinoma. Int J Radiat Oncol Biol Phys 1991;20(1):29–36.

17. Homs MY, Steyerberg EW, Eijkenboom WM, et al. Single-dose brachytherapy versus metal stent placement for the palliation of dysphagia from oesophageal cancer: multicentre randomised trial. Lancet 2004;364(9444):1497–504.
18. Steyerberg EW, Homs MY, Stokvis A, et al. Stent placement or brachytherapy for palliation of dysphagia from esophageal cancer: a prognostic model to guide treatment selection. Gastrointest Endosc 2005;62(3):333–40.
19. Canto M, Smith C, McClelland L, et al. Randomized trial of PDT vs. stent for palliation of malignant dysphagia: cost-effectiveness and quality of life [abstract]. Gastrointest Endsoc 2002;55:100.
20. Dallal HJ, Smith GD, Grieve DC, et al. A randomized trial of thermal ablative therapy versus expandable metal stents in the palliative treatment of patients with esophageal carcinoma. Gastrointest Endosc 2001;54(5):549–57.
21. Conio M, Caroli-Bosc F, Demarquay JF, et al. Self-expanding metal stents in the palliation of neoplasms of the cervical esophagus. Hepatogastroenterology 1999; 46(25):272–7.
22. Eleftheriadis E, Kotzampassi K. Endoprosthesis implantation at the pharyngo-esophageal level: problems, limitations and challenges. World J Gastroenterol 2006;12(13):2103–8.
23. Conio M, Blanchi S, Filiberti R, et al. A modified self-expanding Niti-S stent for the management of benign hypopharyngeal strictures. Gastrointest Endosc 2007; 65(4):714–20.
24. Verschuur EM, Kuipers EJ, Siersema PD. Esophageal stents for malignant strictures close to the upper esophageal sphincter. Gastrointest Endosc 2007;66(6):1082–90.
25. Dua KS, Kozarek R, Kim J, et al. Self-expanding metal esophageal stent with anti-reflux mechanism. Gastrointest Endosc 2001;53(6):603–13.
26. Wenger U, Johnsson E, Arnelo U, et al. An antireflux stent versus conventional stents for palliation of distal esophageal or cardia cancer: a randomized clinical study. Surg Endosc 2006;20(11):1675–80.
27. Homs MY, Wahab PJ, Kuipers EJ, et al. Esophageal stents with antireflux valve for tumors of the distal esophagus and gastric cardia: a randomized trial. Gastrointest Endosc 2004;60(5):695–702.
28. Nishimura Y, Nagata K, Katano S, et al. Severe complications in advanced esophageal cancer treated with radiotherapy after intubation of esophageal stents: a questionnaire survey of the Japanese Society for Esophageal Diseases. Int J Radiat Oncol Biol Phys 2003;56(5):1327–32.
29. Siddiqui AA, Loren D, Dudnick R, et al. Expandable polyester silicon-covered stent for malignant esophageal strictures before neoadjuvant chemoradiation: a pilot study. Dig Dis Sci 2007;52(3):823–9.
30. Siddiqui AA, Glynn C, Loren D, et al. Self-expanding plastic esophageal stents versus jejunostomy tubes for the maintenance of nutrition during neoadjuvant chemoradiation therapy in patients with esophageal cancer: a retrospective study. Dis Esophagus 2009;22(3):216–22.
31. Verschuur EM, Repici A, Kuipers EJ, et al. New design esophageal stents for the palliation of dysphagia from esophageal or gastric cardia cancer: a randomized trial. Am J Gastroenterol 2008;103(2):304–12.
32. Kozarek RA, Ball TJ, Patterson DJ. Metallic self-expanding stent application in the upper gastrointestinal tract: caveats and concerns. Gastrointest Endosc 1992; 38(1):1–6.
33. Dirks K, Schulz T, Schellmann B, et al. Fatal hemorrhage following perforation of the aorta by a barb of the Gianturco-Rosch esophageal stent. Z Gastroenterol 2002;40(2):81–4.

34. Wang MQ, Sze DY, Wang ZP, et al. Delayed complications after esophageal stent placement for treatment of malignant esophageal obstructions and esophagorespiratory fistulas. J Vasc Interv Radiol 2001;12(4):465–74.

35. Baron TH. A practical guide for choosing an expandable metal stent for GI malignancies: is a stent by any other name still a stent? Gastrointest Endosc 2001; 54(2):269–72.

36. Kinsman KJ, DeGregorio BT, Katon RM, et al. Prior radiation and chemotherapy increase the risk of life-threatening complications after insertion of metallic stents for esophagogastric malignancy. Gastrointest Endosc 1996;43(3):196–203.

37. Homs MY, Hansen BE, van Blankenstein M, et al. Prior radiation and/or chemotherapy has no effect on the outcome of metal stent placement for oesophagogastric carcinoma. Eur J Gastroenterol Hepatol 2004;16(2):163–70.

38. Siersema PD, Hop WC, Dees J, et al. Coated self-expanding metal stents versus latex prostheses for esophagogastric cancer with special reference to prior radiation and chemotherapy: a controlled, prospective study. Gastrointest Endosc 1998;47(2):113–20.

39. Homs MY, Siersema PD. Stents in the GI tract. Expert Rev Med Devices 2007; 4(5):741–52.

40. Siersema PD. Endoscopic therapeutic esophageal interventions: what is new? What needs further study? What can we forget? Curr Opin Gastroenterol 2005; 21(4):490–7.

41. Siersema PD. Treatment options for esophageal strictures. Nat Clin Pract Gastroenterol Hepatol 2008;5(3):142–52.

42. Bethge N, Sommer A, Gross U, et al. Human tissue responses to metal stents implanted in vivo for the palliation of malignant stenoses. Gastrointest Endosc 1996;43(6):596–602.

43. Radecke K, Gerken G, Treichel U. Impact of a self-expanding, plastic esophageal stent on various esophageal stenoses, fistulas, and leakages: a single-center experience in 39 patients. Gastrointest Endosc 2005;61(7):812–8.

44. Evrard S, Le Moine O, Lazaraki G, et al. Self-expanding plastic stents for benign esophageal lesions. Gastrointest Endosc 2004;60(6):894–900.

45. Repici A, Conio M, De Angelis C, et al. Temporary placement of an expandable polyester silicone-covered stent for treatment of refractory benign esophageal strictures. Gastrointest Endosc 2004;60(4):513–9.

46. Holm AN, de la Mora Levy JG, Gostout CJ, et al. Self-expanding plastic stents in treatment of benign esophageal conditions. Gastrointest Endosc 2008;67(1):20–5.

47. Karbowski M, Schembre D, Kozarek R, et al. Polyflex self-expanding, removable plastic stents: assessment of treatment efficacy and safety in a variety of benign and malignant conditions of the esophagus. Surg Endosc 2008;22(5):1326–33.

48. Dua KS, Vleggaar FP, Santharam R, et al. Removable self-expanding plastic esophageal stent as a continuous, non-permanent dilator in treating refractory benign esophageal strictures: a prospective two-center study. Am J Gastroenterol 2008;103(12):2988–94.

49. Dua K, Siersema P. Experience with a removal self-expanding plastic esophageal stent (Polyflex Sten) as a continuous, non permanent dilator for refractory benign esophageal strictures [abstract]. Gastrointest Endosc 2007;67(5):148.

50. Sriram PV, Das G, Rao GV, et al. Another novel use of endoscopic clipping: to anchor an esophageal endoprosthesis. Endoscopy 2001;33(8):724–6.

51. Gelbmann CM, Ratiu NL, Rath HC, et al. Use of self-expandable plastic stents for the treatment of esophageal perforations and symptomatic anastomotic leaks. Endoscopy 2004;36(8):695–9.

52. Lee BI, Choi KY, Kang HJ, et al. Sealing an extensive anastomotic leak after esophagojejunostomy with an antimigration-modified covered self-expanding metal stent. Gastrointest Endosc 2006;64(6):1024–6.
53. Ott C, Ratiu N, Endlicher E, et al. Self-expanding Polyflex plastic stents in esophageal disease: various indications, complications, and outcomes. Surg Endosc 2007;21(6):889–96.
54. Eloubeidi MA, Lopes TL. Novel removable internally fully covered self-expanding metal esophageal stent: feasibility, technique of removal, and tissue response in humans. Am J Gastroenterol 2009;104(6):1374–81.
55. Dever J, Schembre D, Brandabur J, et al. Novel use of simultaneous dual endoscopy to reconstitute completely obstructed esophagi and colon [abstract]. Gastrointest Endosc 2009;69(5):230.
56. Price L, Koehler R, Schembre D, et al. The first North American experience with a removable esophageal stent for benign and malignant indications. Am J Gastroenterol, (in press).
57. Brinster CJ, Singhal S, Lee L, et al. Evolving options in the management of esophageal perforation. Ann Thorac Surg 2004;77(4):1475–83.
58. Zumbro GL, Anstadt MP, Mawulawde K, et al. Surgical management of esophageal perforation: role of esophageal conservation in delayed perforation. Am Surg 2002;68(1):36–40.
59. Jougon J, Mc Bride T, Delcambre F, et al. Primary esophageal repair for Boerhaave's syndrome whatever the free interval between perforation and treatment. Eur J Cardiothorac Surg 2004;25(4):475–9.
60. Raju GS, Thompson C, Zwischenberger JB. Emerging endoscopic options in the management of esophageal leaks (videos). Gastrointest Endosc 2005;62(2):278–86.
61. Davies AP, Vaughan R. Expanding mesh stent in the emergency treatment of Boerhaave's syndrome. Ann Thorac Surg 1999;67(5):1482–3.
62. Roy-Choudhury SH, Nicholson AA, Wedgwood KR, et al. Symptomatic malignant gastroesophageal anastomotic leak: management with covered metallic esophageal stents. AJR Am J Roentgenol 2001;176(1):161–5.
63. Siersema PD, Homs MY, Haringsma J, et al. Use of large-diameter metallic stents to seal traumatic nonmalignant perforations of the esophagus. Gastrointest Endosc 2003;58(3):356–61.
64. Chung MG, Kang DH, Park DK, et al. Successful treatment of Boerhaave's syndrome with endoscopic insertion of a self-expandable metallic stent: report of three cases and a review of the literature. Endoscopy 2001;33(10):894–7.
65. Yoon CJ, Shin JH, Song HY, et al. Removal of retrievable esophageal and gastrointestinal stents: experience in 113 patients. AJR Am J Roentgenol 2004;183(5):1437–44.
66. Hasan S, Beckly D, Rahamim J. Oesophagorespiratory fistulas as a complication of self-expanding metal oesophageal stents. Endoscopy 2004;36(8):731–4.
67. Seo YS, Park JJ, Kim BG, et al. Segmental amputation of esophagus with bronchial-wall rupture during removal of a stent for benign esophageal stricture. Gastrointest Endosc 2006;64(1):141–3.
68. Low DE, Kozarek RA. Removal of esophageal expandable metal stents: description of technique and review of potential applications. Surg Endosc 2003;17(6):990–6.
69. Tuncozgur B, Savas MC, Isik AF, et al. Removal of metallic stent by using Polyflex stent in esophago-colic anastomotic stricture. Ann Thorac Surg 2006;82(5):1913–4.

70. Hunerbein M, Stroszczynski C, Moesta KT, et al. Treatment of thoracic anastomotic leaks after esophagectomy with self-expanding plastic stents. Ann Surg 2004;240(5):801–7.
71. Freeman RK, Van Woerkom JM, Ascioti AJ. Esophageal stent placement for the treatment of iatrogenic intrathoracic esophageal perforation. Ann Thorac Surg 2007;83(6):2003–7 [discussion: 2007–8].
72. Petruzziello L, Tringali A, Riccioni ME, et al. Successful early treatment of Boerhaave's syndrome by endoscopic placement of a temporary self-expandable plastic stent without fluoroscopy. Gastrointest Endosc 2003;58(4):608–12.
73. Tuebergen D, Rijcken E, Mennigen R, et al. Treatment of thoracic esophageal anastomotic leaks and esophageal perforations with endoluminal stents: efficacy and current limitations. J Gastrointest Surg 2008;12(7):1168–76.
74. Amrani L, Menard C, Berdah S, et al. From iatrogenic digestive perforation to complete anastomotic disunion: endoscopic stenting as a new concept of "stent-guided regeneration and re-epithelialization". Gastrointest Endosc 2009; 69(7):1282–7.
75. Saito Y, Tanaka T, Andoh A, et al. Usefulness of biodegradable stents constructed of poly-l-lactic acid monofilaments in patients with benign esophageal stenosis. World J Gastroenterol 2007;13(29):3977–80.
76. Seewald S, Ang TL, Omar S, et al. Endoscopic mucosal resection of early esophageal squamous cell cancer using the Duette mucosectomy kit. Endoscopy 2006;38(10):1029–31.
77. Rajan E, Gostout C, Feitoza A, et al. Widespread endoscopic mucosal resection of the esophagus with strategies for stricture prevention: a preclinical study. Endoscopy 2005;37(11):1111–5.
78. Fry SW, Fleischer DE. Management of a refractory benign esophageal stricture with a new biodegradable stent. Gastrointest Endosc 1997;45(2):179–82.
79. Dhar N, Topping J, Johns E, et al. Biodegradable stents in refractory benign oesophageal strictures-first report of 4 patients from the UK. Gastrointest Endosc 2009;69(5):AB254–5.
80. Repici A, Vleggaar F, Calino A, et al. Benign refractory esophageal strictures: preliminary results from the BEST (Biodegradable Esophageal STent) study [abstract]. Gastrointest Endosc 2009;69(5):123.
81. Jeon SR, Eun SH, Shim CS, et al. Effect of drug-eluting metal stents in benign esophageal stricture: an in vivo animal study. Endoscopy 2009;41(5):449–56.
82. De Palma GD, Iovino P, Masone S, et al. Self-expanding metal stents for endoscopic treatment of esophageal achalasia unresponsive to conventional treatments. Long-term results in eight patients. Endoscopy 2001;33(12):1027–30.
83. Hubmann R, Bodlaj G, Czompo M, et al. The use of self-expanding metal stents to treat acute esophageal variceal bleeding. Endoscopy 2006;38(9):896–901.

Natural Orifice Trans-Luminal Endoscopic Surgery in the Esophagus

Timothy A. Woodward, MD[a],*, Laith H. Jamil, MD[b,c],
Michael B. Wallace, MD, MPH[a]

KEYWORDS

- NOTES • Mediastinum • Transesophageal access
- Minimally invasive • Endoscopy

Surgical section of the abdominal wall has been the traditional access to the abdominal cavity and is commonly referred to as open abdominal surgery or laparotomy. Many of the complications of laparotomy that are related to incision of the abdominal wall include incisional pain and extended convalescence, with wound infections occurring in 2% to 25% and incisional hernias in 4% to 18% of patients undergoing laparotomy in the United States.[1,2] The development of laparoscopic surgery has led to smaller incisions, which in turn has led to a marked reduction in incision-related complications.[3] Additionally, a trend toward faster recovery, decreased wound-related infections, and a reduction in postoperative pain have been noted in clinical trials comparing laparoscopic to open procedures.[4,5] Such findings being noted, laparoscopic surgery carries particular risks beyond those of conventional surgery. Procedural complications arise owing to problems with maneuverability and visualization, and the lack of tactile feedback in a 2-dimensional visual field imposes limitations not manifest in classic open procedures.[6,7] Complications arise from injuries to vascular structures via needles and trochars; carbon dioxide gas emboli can occur from the creation of a pneumoperitoneum. Injury rates up to three times that of laparotomy had, at one time, been reported.[8–10] Although the rates of complications have been reduced over recent years,[11] this history should be kept in mind as we embark again upon new surgical procedures.

This work was supported by Coviden Award of the American Society for Gastrointestinal Endoscopy (ASGE).

[a] Division of Gastroenterology, Mayo Clinic College of Medicine, 4500 San Pablo Road, Jacksonville, FL 32224, USA
[b] David Geffen School of Medicine at UCLA, Los Angeles, CA, USA
[c] Cedars-Sinai Medical Center, Los Angeles, CA, USA
* Corresponding author.
E-mail address: woodward.timothy@mayo.edu (T.A. Woodward).

Natural orifice transluminal endoscopic surgery (NOTES) is part of the spectrum of evolving surgical concepts. The idea of endoscopic manipulations taking place outside the gastrointestinal lumen was validated with the success of procedures such as the endoscopic transgastric pseudocyst drainage,[12] or the transesophageal management of mediastinal abscesses.[13] Reports such as the complete removal of a necrotic spleen by transgastric debridement,[14] as well as pancreatic necrosectomy,[15] give weight to therapeutic endoscopic endeavors proceeding beyond simple biopsies and aspirates. Additionally, the surprisingly low incidence of complications after accidental puncture with immediate closure of the gastric wall with endoscopic tumor removal[16] or large colonic polypectomies[17] supported the resolve of endoscopic researchers to perform endoscopic surgery via a natural orifice.

NOTES involves the insertion of flexible endoscopes through natural orifices such as the mouth, rectum, or vagina, with the subsequent incision and penetration of the lumen to gain access to surrounding structures. There are hypothetical benefits of NOTES over conventional open and laparoscopic surgery. The absence of a surface incision eliminates cutaneous scarring and infection[18]; anesthesia and analgesia requirements can be decreased[19] along with a reduction in recovery time,[20] and hernia and adhesions formation.[21,22] Morbidly obese patients may undergo intra-abdominal surgeries that were previously inadvisable by cutaneous incision.[23] Finally, economically impoverished countries, where traditional surgical access may be limited and untenable, may now have a viable option for operative care (C. Smith, personal communication, 2008).

As with the introduction of laparoscopic surgery, issues of visualization, orientation, access, and manipulation still need to be addressed before NOTES surgery can be feasible. A number of intra-abdominal NOTES studies have been undertaken to evaluate models, techniques, outcomes, and clinical applicability. A recent review examined 34 intra-abdominal NOTES experimental studies.[24] Of these, 30 were animal based, thus limiting evidence-based interpretations. Of the four human clinical studies, only two represent a series. Hazey and colleagues' study[25] was a comparison between NOTES peritoneoscopy with diagnostic laparoscopy in 10 patients with a pancreatic mass. Peritoneal access was obtained via an anterior transgastric approach with a mean exploration time of 24 minutes (compared with 13 minutes for laparoscopic evaluation). The decision to proceed with open exploration was consistent for both in 90% (9 of 10 cases); however, in comparison with laparoscopic, 40% visualization of the right lobe of the liver and right upper quadrant structures was inadequate using NOTES. Tsin and colleagues' study[26] was a case series of 100 patients using a hybrid of mini-laparoscopic–assisted natural orifice surgery for benign surgical conditions. Finally, with animal studies, although intra-abdominal access could be achieved, the best route and method still has not been established.[24] Site closure could not be achieved in all cases and risk of peritoneal infection could not be adequately minimized.[24]

As limited as are the studies regarding peritoneal NOTES, mediastinal transluminal experiments are certainly in their infancy. We evaluate, in this review, the parallel development of minimally invasive thoracic surgery with regard to its counterpart in peritoneal laparoscopy to NOTES. Transesophageal interventions by both endosonographic and direct visualization are examined in the context of minimally invasive surgery and mediastinal NOTES. Techniques of viscerotomy creation (ie, formation of access routes), visualization, and closure are examined with particular emphasis on mediastinal structures. The state of current interventions is examined. Finally, current morbidity (including infectious complications) and survival outcomes are examined in those animals that have undergone transesophageal exploration.

MINIMALLY INVASIVE CHEST SURGERY

In 1866, *The Dublin Journal of Medical Science* published a report entitled "Most extensive pleuritic effusion rapidly becoming purulent, paracentesis, introduction of a drainage tube, recovery, examination of interior of pleura by the endoscope." The article reported the use of a "new endoscope" developed by a Dr. Francis Richard Cruise in which he performed a thoracoscopy on an 11-year-old girl with an infected pleural cavity.[27]

There have evolved, since the first published reports in the nineteenth century, techniques to visualize the mediastinum that coincide with laparoscopic technological innovation. Mediastinoscopy is a minimally invasive procedure that allows visualization of thoracic lymph node stations 2, 3, 4, 7, and 10 in the staging of lung cancers.[28] To visualize stations 5 and 6, thoracic surgeons use an anterior mediastinotomy (Chamberlain procedure) to access these nodes.[28] Over the past decade, video mediastinoscopy has progressed to allow for much better visualization of the mediastinum to facilitate lymph node sampling.[29] In experienced hands, video mediastinoscopy provides better visualization of the mediastinum, allowing the surgeon to visualize structures that are normally not seen, such as the recurrent laryngeal nerves and the esophagus.[30]

Video-assisted thoracoscopic surgery (VATS) has demonstrable advantages over the traditional thoracotomy, particularly for lung cancer. VATS allows for a small, muscle-sparing incision that allows for visualization of the thorax without spreading the ribs. First described in the early 1990s as a technique in the resection of lung cancer,[31,32] the literature has shown significant short-term advantages of VATS lobectomy, with recent findings demonstrating long-term oncologic outcomes for VATS similar to traditional open resections.[33] Perioperative mortality rates are low, between 0.5% and 2.7% with low conversion rates in the largest series.[34-36] The most common complications of arrhythmias, pneumonia, air leak, and myocardial infarction are similar to those reported in the open literature.[37] Short-term outcomes after VATS lobectomy include, as in laparoscopic surgery, low operative blood loss,[38] less postoperative pain,[39] and a quicker return to baseline function.[40] Additionally, 12 months after surgery, none of the patients in Sugiura and colleagues[38] study who had undergone VATS lobectomy complained of post-thoracotomy pain, whereas 26.7% of those undergoing traditional thoracotomy were still taking narcotics for chest pain. Key, however, are the long-term oncologic outcomes. Onaitis and colleagues[34] in a cohort of 500 patients demonstrated a 2-year survival rate for stage 1 and stage 2 disease of 85% and 77%. A randomized trial of 100 patients with 1A lung cancer demonstrated no significant difference in 3- and 5-year overall survival rates between the two groups.[33]

In 1994 a report by McAnena and colleagues[41] described a thoracoscopic-assisted mobilization combined with an open abdominal approach for esophageal resection. A year later, DePaula and colleagues[42] demonstrated the feasibility of laparoscopic transhiatal esophagectomy. From thence, there have been a myriad of minimally invasive esophagectomy (MIE) approaches, which include thoracoscopic-assisted esophageal resection and combined thoracoscopic-laparoscopic resection.[43,44] Regardless of the approach, safety and feasibility of minimally invasive esophagectomy are equivalent to traditional open approaches. Nguyen and colleagues[45] demonstrated, using a combined thoracoscopic-laparoscopic approach, a mortality (4.3%), major complication (17.4%), and anastomotic leak (8.7%) equivalent to historic controls.[46] Luketich and colleagues[47] have reported the largest series to date of MIE. Again, using a combined approach, 222 patients demonstrated 30-day mortality and anastomotic leak rates similar to historical series with a mean hospital stay of 7 days, much less than seen in open series. Regarding the oncologic adequacy of MIE, several case series suggest outcomes that are comparable with open. Braghetto and colleagues[48] reported a consecutive series of 166 patients undergoing MIE for esophageal cancer. Three-year survival rates were 93.8% for stage 1 disease and 54% for stage 2a disease; there was no significant difference when compared with the open group.

Thus, current data support the use of thoracoscopic techniques with improved short-term outcomes related to a decrease in postoperative pain, less blood loss, and shorter length hospital stay. Studies have demonstrated an immunologic benefit with VATS, resulting in decreased cytokine release and improved lymphocyte function,[49,50] and there is a return to preoperative function that is related to the avoidance of rib-spreading thoracotomy.[51] However, transesophageal mediastinoscopy and thoracoscopy could eliminate chest wall trauma, for even with a small incision, pain and a relatively extended hospital stay are significant.[52,53]

ENDOSCOPY AND MINIMALLY INVASIVE ASSESSMENT OF AND ACCESS TO THE MEDIASTINUM

Endoscopists have used endoscopic ultrasound (EUS) to image and access the mediastinum for a number of years.[54–56] EUS-guided techniques allow for comprehensive assessment of the mediastinum in the staging of lung cancers. Mediastinal lymph nodes are the most common site of metastases. Patients without evidence of mediastinal lymph node involvement are offered surgical resection, whereas those with lymph node involvement are potentially offered neoadjuvant treatment.[57] Mediastinoscopy, as noted above, is a minimally invasive surgical procedure that is considered the diagnostic standard, but it has limitations.[58] Mediastinoscopy allows for only limited access to the inferior and posterior mediastinum and aortopulmonary window.[59] EUS fine-needle aspirate (EUS-FNA) has emerged over the past decade as a valuable tool in the mediastinal staging of lung cancers. Using the real-time capabilities of sector scanning that allow for direct visualization of the needle as it passes through the esophageal wall, direct aspirate of adjacent lymph nodes can be undertaken.[60] Direct comparisons between EUS and mediastinoscopy are few; however, in a trial by Larsen and colleagues,[61] which compared EUS-FNA with mediastinoscopy in patients with paratracheal or subcarinal lymphadenopathy, EUS-FNA was significantly more accurate than mediastinoscopy in the subcarina. Endobronchial ultrasound (EBUS) with FNA complements the mediastinal access of EUS-FNA. EBUS-FNA is able to assess the anterior mediastinum.[62] The combination of the two may supplant mediastinoscopy in some instances of lung cancer staging, as demonstrated by our study.[63] Of 138 patients, the combination of EUS-FNA and EBUS-FNA had an estimated sensitivity of 93% and a negative predictive value of 97% in detecting lymph nodes in any mediastinal location.

Beyond mediastinal FNA, endosonography has been used in the management of paraesophageal abscesses. Nonoperative management of esophageal perforation and its sequelae is acceptable in select patients with well-contained perforation and minimal mediastinal soilage. There are criteria for nonoperative management[64,65]: an early or well-circumscribed perforation; a non-neoplastic esophageal disruption that is contained within the mediastinum; drainage of the cavity into the esophagus; and minimal signs of clinical sepsis. The first reported use of endoscopy to access mediastinal fluid collections was by Kanshin and Pogodina in 1983,[66] in which they described the first successful endoscopic transesophageal insertion of a nasomediastinal drain. This technique was later complemented by Abe and colleagues,[67] who described the successful nasomediastinal drain insertion and closure of an esophageal perforation after foreign-body-related mediastinitis. EUS has led to the ability to visualize the mediastinum and allow insertion of catheters and stents for drainage.[68] Drains cannot manage necrotic debris, and some circumstances warrant necrosectomy as well as irrigation. Wehrmann and colleagues[13] had expanded the endoscopic and EUS-guided interventions with direct endoscopic debridement. Using strategies developed in the aggressive management of peripancreatic necrosis by way of transgastric endoscopy and debridement,[69] 20 patients were treated with EUS-guided or endoscopic mediastinal puncture for abscesses greater than 2 cm. None of the patients had responded to conservative management prior, which was, by definition, an indication for traditional surgery. Abscesses were entered with a 9.5-mm endoscope after balloon dilation to allow irrigation and drainage. Debris was removed with a Dormia basket. Debridement was successful in all cases, although a median of five daily sessions was required.

EUS has evolved into a valuable adjunct in NOTES applications with several investigators demonstrating the benefits of endosonographic visualization. Chak and colleagues[70] have shown, for example, in a porcine model, the utility of EUS in the initial NOTES incision. NOTES incisions were made in the rectum, the posterior gastric wall, and the gastric antrum at 16 locations defined as safe (no vessel or organ adjacent to the wall) and 16 locations defined as unsafe. Incisions made in locations defined as safe were generally safe, except for three rectal incisions that resulted in small bowel injuries. All unsafe incisions resulted in major injuries such as gallbladder perforation, liver laceration, arterial bleeding, and death. In addition to its potential role in guiding the initial incision, other applications in animal models have been explored using EUS in NOTES. These include tissue apposition, gastrojejunostomy, lymphnode dissection, gastropexy, and cardiac catherization.[71–75]

MEDIASTINAL NOTES

The techniques used for a transesophageal approach for debridement of mediastinal abscesses may be expanded to explore the mediastinum. However, unlike its peritoneal counterpart, the platform for exploration mediastinal NOTES is, paradoxically, somewhat limited by its relative simplicity. Whereas entrance to the peritoneum can be made by a transvesical, transcolon, transvaginal, or transgastric approach, the esophagus provides the only natural orifice with access to the mediastinum. The posterior mediastinum is delimited by critical structures such as the descending thoracic aorta, the esophagus, the azygos vein, and the autonomic ganglia and nerves. In addition, as a straight tubular structure, direction and navigation through the esophagus is limited. Thus, the point of entrance into the mediastinum is paramount. In our studies, using EUS to guide entrance sites allowed for right-sided, atraumatic needle-knife incisions at both subcarinal and aortic arch locations,[76] with the aortic arch entrance allowing for antegrade, ie, forward-viewing exploration and intervention. This, in our opinion, is preferred over an entrance point that requires retroflex manipulation for certain structures. Additionally, we have found that having the animal in the left lateral decubitus position (versus supine) allows for better mechanical ventilation and subsequent oxygenation of the pig.

NOTES Mediastinal Viscerotomy

Irrespective of the point of entrance, the proximity of pulmonary and cardiovascular structures over the course of the mediastinum place premium importance on the type of initial incision that is made. Concerns regarding infection and bleeding, closure, and healing of the incision site have led to various approaches to the opening cut. In most transgastric studies, gastrotomies were created with a needle knife to make the initial gastric incision, with subsequent enlargement with a dilation balloon.[14,72,77,78] Subsequent studies use a sphincterotome to enlarge the incision, with the advantage obtained of speed and access for repeated passage.[79] Most mediastinal NOTES studies use a mucosal flap safety valve in an effort to provide a mucosal seal. The overlying esophageal mucosa is used to control contamination from a perforating muscle layer resection. Sumiyama and colleagues[80] describe a technique by which a mucosal flap valve is created. Initially, a bleb of saline solution is injected to confirm placement of the needle tip into the submucosa, followed by a millisecond burst of high-pressure carbon dioxide. Subsequently, a biliary retrieval balloon was used to expand the submucosal space. Distal to the mucosal entry point and within the submucosal tunneled space, the muscularis propria is penetrated to enter the mediastinum. We have used a similar method to enter the submucosal space by adapting a technique from endoscopic mucosal resection. Hydroxypropylmethylcellulose is injected to dissect the submucosal connective tissue, followed by extension of the expansion by insufflation of a biliary balloon.[76] Other groups have used esophageal bands to remove the mucosa, exposing the muscularis propria; this is followed by blunt dissection of the exposed submucosal space with the snare tip.[81] In most of the animal models, a needle knife penetrates the muscularis propria, creating an offset entrance into the mediastinum by way of an overlying mucosal flap; the mucosal entry point may thus be closed with an endoscopic clip or a tissue anchoring system. Sumiyama and colleagues,[80] using an endoscopic mucosal resection cap, create a muscularis propria defect through an aspiration myotomy; hypothetically, this approach would eliminate inadvertent injury to surrounding structures in the mediastinum. Regardless of how the tunnel is created, creating a submucosal flap, by burrowing 10 to 15 cm from the distal exit through the muscular portion of the esophageal wall, allows for mucosal approximation that may prevent postprocedural leaks.

Of concern is the eventual strength of the defect created in the esophageal wall. Fritscher-Ravens and colleagues[82] examined the incision site, macroscopically as well as histologically, several weeks after esophageal wall closure. Using a suturing system, they were able to create a full-thickness approximation of the wall with, subsequently, a full-thickness scar. However, when clip closure was used there was histologically demonstrated closure of only the mucosal defect; the muscular layer was intermittently incomplete. Although the seal was overall intact, there is the hypothetical concern of a persistent weakness in the esophageal wall, leading to diverticula. It should be noted that the porcine esophagus is composed of only a striated muscle layer in the lower esophagus, whereas the human esophagus consists of an outer longitudinal and inner circular layer of smooth muscle. Thus, animal findings may not be representative of what happens with humans. Additionally, the mucosal flap technique mirrors the muscular layer changes in the Heller myotomy with a mucosal flap overlying the myotomy. Clinical practice thus offers some indirect reassurance of the integrity of the wall postincision. In addition, also as seen from clinical practice, temporary placement of an esophageal stent over the defect may present an option to suture or clip closure.[83]

NOTES Mediastinal Visualization

With a transesophageal window, entrance is into the posterior compartment of the mediastinum. Using only an endoscopic view, it can be difficult to ascertain the safety of the entrance site. As previously noted, EUS facilitates an appropriate entrance.[84] At approximately 35 cm from the porcine snout, the aortic arch is identified. Rotation of the scope clockwise 25 degrees allowed for visualization and entrance into a right-sided vessel-free space (**Fig. 1**A and B). A site is marked with an injection of methylene blue by a 19-gauge EUS needle, 6 to 10 cm above the aortic arch, with subsequent re-intubation by a standard upper endoscope. A submucosal tunnel is created from the marked site. Entrance and dissection can be facilitated by a tapered cap and needle-knife. The submucosal space is characterized by web-like connective tissue and a paucity of vessels. Crucial, however, is maintaining orientation, as extended tunnels may inadvertently shift from the targeted entrance point.

Upon entering the mediastinum, discontinuing endoscopic insufflation is of benefit to prevent tension pneumothorax and tension pneumomediastinum.[81] CO_2 is also a consideration if insufflation is necessary in exploration.[24] Entrance into the mediastinal compartment to the right of the aortic arch allows visualization of the descending thoracic aorta, the exterior esophagus, hilar lymph nodes, pleura, lung, and left and right vagus nerves. Additionally, we have found that establishing the entrance above the aortic arch, to the thoracic inlet allows for the additional visualization of the trachea and potentially branches of the vagus, as well as the aforementioned structures, in an antegrade orientation. With entrance into the mediastinum, left/right orientation is sometimes difficult to maintain, as the single site access does not allow for a secondary point for fixation; antegrade visualization is helpful in this regard. We, and other groups, have used a video-assisted thoracoscope in our initial studies to ascertain accuracy regarding structures that are identified and orientation.

With extension, the thoracic cavity may be accessed as well. Transesophageal thoracoscopy is accomplished with the creation of a small tear through the pleura with endoscopic forceps. Transesophageal thoracoscopy allows for identification of the lung, the pleura, pericardium, and the superior surface of the diaphragm. With entrance into the pleural space, care must be taken that overinsufflation does not lead to a pneumothorax. Use of selective intubation of the contralateral lung and collapse of the ipsilateral lung may prevent this complication (S. Aniskevich, personal communication, 2008).

Mediastinal NOTES Intervention and Techniques

Lymphadenectomy

First reports with mediastinal NOTES demonstrated the ease by which lymph nodes could be accessed via a transesophageal approach **Fig. 2**.[76,82,85] Lymph node resection was accomplished using endoscopic biopsy forceps. Fritscher-Ravens and colleagues[73] used EUS to detect small mediastinal lymph nodes in two pigs. Small lymph nodes can be difficult to detect in that they can be imbedded in fatty tissue. By fixing the lymph nodes with a threaded anchor, the tissue and nodes were identified and subsequently removed by polypectomy snare.

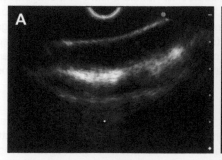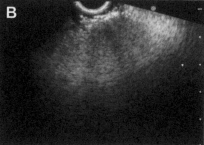

Fig. 1. (A) Porcine aortic arch. (B) Right-sided vessel-free space.

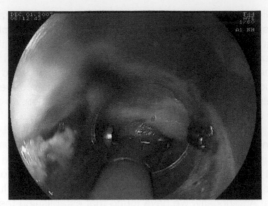

Fig. 2. Subcarinal lymphadenectomy.

Pleural biopsy

As noted earlier, the pleura is easy to access transesophageally but is somewhat fibrous, requiring a little more force for biopsy by endoscopic forceps. A major advantage of the transesophageal approach is that direct visualization allows for full assessment of the thoracic cavity, particularly with regard to the central area. This would present a distinct advantage over blind percutaneous pleural biopsy. In a survival series of three pigs, Rattner and colleagues performed pleural biopsies with necropsies done at 8 to 12 days.[81] Only mild atelectasis was found as a minimal complication. This was felt secondary to transient desaturation and possibly prolonged anesthesia recovery.

Pericardial/cardiac access

Fritscher-Ravens and colleagues,[82] in their survival animal series, performed, in five pigs, a superficial incision into the pericardium for fenestration. In four animals, saline was injected into the myocardium. Both procedures were well tolerated. Necropsy at 4 weeks revealed no pericarditis.

Gostout and colleagues have reported, on a series of five pigs, their experience by which the heart was evaluated transesophageally.[86] After the mucosa of the esophagus was cleansed with povidone-iodine via the endoscope channel, a submucosal tunnel was created with subsequent access to the posterior mediastinum. Following a pleural incision with a hook needle knife, the pleural cavity was entered. Following visualization of the heart, a pericardial puncture was undertaken, followed by the creation of a 3-cm pericardial window via an insulated-tip needle-knife. Point coagulation was performed on the epicardium through the pericardial window using a heat probe and hook-knife. The procedure was performed in 30 minutes in four of the five pigs (one pig sustained inadvertent injury to the descending aorta) with no sustained cardiac rhythm changes. Follow-up endoscopy a week later revealed a healed mucosal entry site; necropsy revealed patency of all pericardial windows with no cardiac abnormalities present.

Vagotomy

Upon entrance into the mediastinum, blunt dissection around the esophagus with either the endoscope or balloon dilator exposes both the left and right vagus nerves. In our nonsurvival study,[76] the vagus was isolated in six pigs with subsequent vagotomy by hot biopsy forceps **Fig. 3**. Necropsy performed on two of the pigs revealed no areas of injury adjacent to the thermal vagotomy.

Spinal interventions
Certain select spine surgeries are performed via a thoracoscopic access, eg, thoracoscopic sympathectomy. The proximity of the esophagus to the anterior thoracic spine favors a transesophageal approach. Kalloo and colleagues[87] proceeded to identify the technical challenges set forth from a NOTES approach. Four pigs underwent endoscopic evaluation of the posterior mediastinum. The pigs were changed to a prone position for better visualization of the thoracic spine. After mediastinoscopy, 5-mm incisions were performed in the anterior longitudinal ligament using a needle-knife at the level of the proximal, middle, and distal thoracic spine. A 19-gauge needle was advanced into the vertebral body and intervertebral space under fluoroscopic monitoring. Bone biopsy was performed using a 19-gauge needle or biopsy forceps. The pigs were immediately euthanized with the procedure demonstrating a cut of approximately 1 cm into the three vertebral bodies while avoiding adjacent structures. This approach may allow for intervertebral interventions with relative ease and safety.

Submucosal esophageal myotomy
An endoscopic approach to achalasia has been hampered by the risk of perforation as the mucosal layer is incised through to the muscular layer. As surmised, the availability of a mucosal flap by way of the submucosal tunnel in the esophagus allows for a potentially safe and effective method of myotomy **Fig. 4**. Pasricha and colleagues, in four pigs, entered 5 cm above the lower esophageal sphincter (LES), and after creating a submucosal space with a 12-mm dilation balloon, tunneled toward the visible muscular layer of the LES. Using a needle-knife, the circular muscle layer was incised in a distal-to-proximal manner without complications. Manometry was performed and the pigs were killed after 5 to 7 days, with a demonstrable decrease in the LES pressures.[88] Necropsy revealed no evidence of mediastinitis and the outermost esophageal wall was intact in all animals.

Assistance in minimally invasive esophagectomy
The next generation of NOTES therapeutics has emphasized more pragmatic use of endoscopy as an adjunct to thoracoscopic or laparoscopic procedures. Evolving from our mediastinal studies are methods in which transesophageal dissection of the esophagus may facilitate minimally invasive esophagectomy.[89] With five pigs,

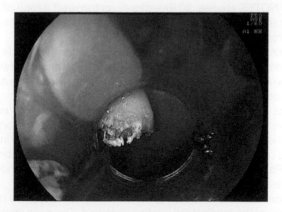

Fig. 3. Vagotomy.

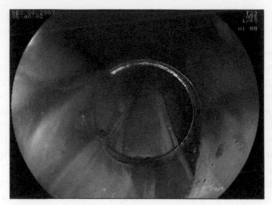

Fig. 4. Esophagomyotomy.

a site was chosen on the right-lateral wall of the esophagus as a transesophageal entry site into the mediastinum (first determined by EUS; later by transillumination); a 10-mL superior mediastinal access site with mucosal flap in the region of the thoracic inlet/aortic arch was created with a needle-knife following the injection of Gonak solution (hydroxypropyl methylcellulose) to facilitate tunneling. From this vantage point, we were able to visualize the trachea, anterior indentation of the thoracic spine, posterior aorta, and both branches of the vagus. Repeated insufflation of the biliary balloon allowed for bloodless dissection of surrounding structures along with the needle-knife. Eventual 360-degree mobilization of the esophagus was accomplished from the entrance point down to the diaphragmatic hiatus. The pigs were immediately humanely killed for necropsy whereupon it was ascertained that visualization of the mediastinum and circumferential mobilization of the esophagus were obtainable via a superior mediastinal approach. Structures and vessels could be easily identified and dissection in the antegrade manner was undertaken. The study demonstrated that transesophageal access to the mediastinum can potentially accomplish good exposure for mediastinal dissection of the esophagus, particularly given that the endoluminal access site would be removed with the specimen.

Safety

Of the peritoneal NOTES studies, 20 investigations followed a total of 109 animals for survival periods ranging from 1 to 28 days,[24] with mortality ranging from 0% to 67% (median: 0%) across 20 studies.

Of the mediastinal NOTES survival studies reviewed for this article,[80–82,88,90] there were only three deaths reported. All were procedure related with two secondary to respiratory compromise following injury to the pleura; one was attributable to inadvertent injury to the aorta.

Survival periods ranged from 8 to 28 days. Surprisingly, although one report found mild atelectasis in 75% of the pigs at necropsy, there were no reported episodes of mediastinal infection or viscerotomy failure. There was one reported instance of an intramural abscess manifesting as contained fluid collection in the submucosal esophageal tunnel.[81] Pathologic evaluation revealed bacteria and abundant neutrophils suggesting abscess formation.

Incidental, procedure-related bleeding (ie, small vessel bleed) was not documented as a problem in any of the mediastinal studies reviewed. The main complications in our experience as well as that sited by other investigators, is the inadvertent injury to the pleura, resulting in respiratory compromise and incisional injury to the aorta with the needle-knife (Woodward T, Wallace M, Raimondo M, personal communication, 2008).

Although the limited array of procedures demonstrate the technical feasibility of performing transesophageal interventions, these procedures have yet to be optimized for effectiveness and minimization of risk.

Future Directions

As with its peritoneal counterpart, mediastinal NOTES is a multidisciplinary endeavor involving gastroenterologists and thoracic surgery. However, the consensus statement from the Natural Orifice Surgery Consortium for Assessment and Research (NO-SCAR) group still is applicable to our mediastinal ventures, ie, "NOTES is truly surgery and should be developed and promoted by surgeons, knowledgeable in suturing, wound healing, anatomy and other surgical options."[91–93] With refinement of the technical challenges facilitated by transesophageal procedures, prospective comparative studies need to be undertaken between mediastinal NOTES and its thoracoscopic/VATS counterpart. More intriguing is the development of hybrid studies (ie, VATS/transesophageal) that could serve as a bridge to early human clinical procedures. For example, transesophageal lymph node mapping and resection could complement staging with the added benefit of excising whole nodes as compared with EUS/FNA as well biopsy of lesions not accessible without a minithoracotomy.[94]

Conclusion

There is much that is intellectually appealing regarding mediastinal NOTES. The elimination of chest wall trauma is an attractive prospect. Ready access to difficult to reach compartments of the mediastinum, makes a transesophageal approach a welcome addition to the procedural repertoire. There are several difficulties, however, that may limit mediastinal NOTES at present. First, arguably more so than the peritoneum, the mediastinum is an unforgiving space, both from the standpoint of the major structures that inhabit the area as well as the devastating morbidity associated with mediastinitis. In addition, the data presented by the studies done so far are limited by sample size, restricting the data interpretation to case-report analyses. Future studies will need to compare NOTES procedures to standard surgical intervention as we move from the developmental to the clinical stage.

SUMMARY

There is much that is intellectually appealing to the application of NOTES procedures to the mediastinum. The elimination of chest wall trauma as well as ready access to hard-to-reach compartments of the mediastinum make a transesophageal approach a welcome addition to the procedural repertoire. As limited as are the studies regarding peritoneal NOTES, however, mediastinal transluminal experiments are in their infancy. We evaluated, in this review, transesophageal interventions within the context of the current animal models that are available.

REFERENCES

1. McGee MF, Rosen MJ, Marks J, et al. A primer on natural orifice transluminal endoscopic surgery: building a new paradigm. Surg Innov 2006;13(2):86–93.
2. Boni L, Benevento A, Rovera F, et al. Infective complications in laparoscopic surgery. Surg Infect (Larchmt) 2006;7(Suppl 2):S109–11.

3. Sauerland S, Lefering R, Neugebauer E. Laprascopic versus open surgery for suspected appendicitis. Cochrane Database Syst Rev 2004;(4):CD001546.
4. Kapischke M, Caliebe A, Tepel J, et al. Open versus laparoscopic appendicectomy: a critical review. Surg Endosc 2006;20(7):1060–8.
5. Calland JF, Tanaka K, Foley E, et al. Outpatient laparoscopic cholecystectomy: patient outcomes after implementation of a clinical pathway. Ann Surg 2001; 233(5):704–15.
6. Osborne DA, Alexander G, Boe B, et al. Laparoscopic cholecystectomy: past, present, and future. Surg Technol Int 2006;15:81–5.
7. Wolf JS Jr. Devices for hand-assisted laparoscopic surgery. Expert Rev Med Devices 2005;2(6):725–30.
8. Johnson WR. Laparoscopic surgery: time for re-evaluation. Med J Aust 1996; 165(7):355–6.
9. Lau WY, Leow CK, Li AK. History of endoscopic and laparoscopic surgery. World J Surg 1997;21(4):444–53.
10. Slim K, Bousquet J, Kwiatkowski F, et al. Analysis of randomized controlled trials in laparoscopic surgery. Br J Surg 1997;84(5):610–4.
11. Fuchs KH. Minimally invasive surgery. Endoscopy 2002;34(2):154–9.
12. Baron TH. Endoscopic drainage of pancreatic fluid collections and pancreatic necrosis. Gastrointest Endosc Clin N Am 2003;13(4):743–64.
13. Wehrmann T, Stergiou N, Vogel B, et al. Endoscopic debridement of paraesophageal, mediastinal abscesses: a prospective case series. Gastrointest Endosc 2005;62(3):344–9.
14. Kantsevoy SV, Hu B, Jagannath SB, et al. Transgastric endoscopic splenectomy: is it possible? Surg Endosc 2006;20(3):522–5.
15. Seifert H, Wehrmann T, Schmitt T, et al. Retroperitoneal endoscopic debridement for infected peripancreatic necrosis. Lancet 2000;356(9230):653–5.
16. Isomoto H, Shikuwa S, Yamaguchi N, et al. Endoscopic submucosal dissection for early gastric cancer: a large-scale feasibility study. Gut 2009;58(3):331–6.
17. Hurlstone DP, Sanders DS, Cross SS, et al. Colonoscopic resection of lateral spreading tumours: a prospective analysis of endoscopic mucosal resection. Gut 2004;53(9):1334–9.
18. ASGE/SAGES. ASGE/SAGES Working Group on Natural Orifice Translumenal Endoscopic Surgery White Paper October 2005. Gastrointest Endosc 2006; 63(2):199–203.
19. Ekstein P, Szold A, Sagie B, et al. Laparoscopic surgery may be associated with severe pain and high analgesia requirements in the immediate postoperative period. Ann Surg 2006;243(1):41–6.
20. Giday SA, Kantsevoy SV, Kalloo AN. Principle and history of Natural Orifice Translumenal Endoscopic Surgery (NOTES). Minim Invasive Ther Allied Technol 2006; 15(6):373–7.
21. Kalloo AN, Singh VK, Jagannath SB, et al. Flexible transgastric peritoneoscopy: a novel approach to diagnostic and therapeutic interventions in the peritoneal cavity. Gastrointest Endosc 2004;60(1):114–7.
22. Hochberger J, Lamade W. Transgastric surgery in the abdomen: the dawn of a new era? Gastrointest Endosc 2005;62(2):293–6.
23. Alexander JW. Wound infections in the morbidly obese. Obes Surg 2005;15(9): 1276–7.
24. Flora ED, Wilson TG, Martin IJ, et al. A review of natural orifice translumenal endoscopic surgery (NOTES) for intra-abdominal surgery: experimental models, techniques, and applicability to the clinical setting. Ann Surg 2008;247(4):583–602.

25. Hazey JW, Narula VK, Renton DB, et al. Natural-orifice transgastric endo-scopic peritoneoscopy in humans: initial clinical trial. Surg Endosc 2008; 22(1):16–20.
26. Tsin DA, Colombero LT, Lambeck J, et al. Minilaparoscopy-assisted natural orifice surgery. JSLS 2007;11(1):24–9.
27. Solli P, Spaggiari L. Indications and developments of video-assisted thoracic surgery in the treatment of lung cancer. Oncologist 2007;12(10):1205–14.
28. Detterbeck FC, DeCamp MM Jr, Kohman LJ, et al. Lung cancer. Invasive staging: the guidelines. Chest 2003;123(1 Suppl):167S–75S.
29. Lin J, Iannettoni MD. The role of thoracoscopy in the management of lung cancer. Surg Oncol 2003;12(3):195–200.
30. Murasugi M, Onuki T, Ikeda T, et al. The role of video-assisted thoracoscopic surgery in the diagnosis of the small peripheral pulmonary nodule. Surg Endosc 2001;15(7):734–6.
31. McKenna R Jr. Vats lobectomy with mediastinal lymph node sampling or dissec-tion. Chest Surg Clin N Am 1995;5(2):223–32.
32. D'Amico TA. Thoracoscopic lobectomy: evolving and improving. J Thorac Cardi-ovasc Surg 2006;132(3):464–5.
33. Sugi K, Kaneda Y, Esato K. Video-assisted thoracoscopic lobectomy achieves a satisfactory long-term prognosis in patients with clinical stage IA lung cancer. World J Surg 2000;24(1):27–30 [discussion: 30–1].
34. Onaitis MW, Petersen RP, Balderson SS, et al. Thoracoscopic lobectomy is a safe and versatile procedure: experience with 500 consecutive patients. Ann Surg 2006;244(3):420–5.
35. Swanson SJ, Herndon JE 2nd, D'Amico TA, et al. Video-assisted thoracic surgery lobectomy: report of CALGB 39802–a prospective, multi-institution feasibility study. J Clin Oncol 2007;25(31):4993–7.
36. Roviaro G, Varoli F, Vergani C, et al. Long-term survival after videothoracoscopic lobectomy for stage I lung cancer. Chest 2004;126(3):725–32.
37. Choh MS, Madura JA 2nd. The role of minimally invasive treatments in surgical oncology. Surg Clin North Am 2009;89(1):53–77, viii.
38. Sugiura H, Morikawa T, Kaji M, et al. Long-term benefits for the quality of life after video-assisted thoracoscopic lobectomy in patients with lung cancer. Surg Lap-arosc Endosc Percutan Tech 1999;9(6):403–8.
39. Giudicelli R, Thomas P, Lonjon T, et al. Video-assisted minithoracotomy versus muscle-sparing thoracotomy for performing lobectomy. Ann Thorac Surg 1994; 58(3):712–7 [discussion: 17–8].
40. Landreneau RJ, Hazelrigg SR, Mack MJ, et al. Postoperative pain-related morbidity: video-assisted thoracic surgery versus thoracotomy. Ann Thorac Surg 1993;56(6):1285–9.
41. McAnena OJ, Rogers J, Williams NS. Right thoracoscopically assisted oesopha-gectomy for cancer. Br J Surg 1994;81(2):236–8.
42. DePaula AL, Hashiba K, Ferreira EA, et al. Laparoscopic transhiatal esophagec-tomy with esophagogastroplasty. Surg Laparosc Endosc 1995;5(1):1–5.
43. Bonavina L, Bona D, Binyom PR, et al. A laparoscopy-assisted surgical approach to esophageal carcinoma. J Surg Res 2004;117(1):52–7.
44. Smithers BM, Gotley DC, McEwan D, et al. Thoracoscopic mobilization of the esophagus. A 6 year experience. Surg Endosc 2001;15(2):176–82.
45. Nguyen NT, Roberts P, Follette DM, et al. Thoracoscopic and laparoscopic esophagectomy for benign and malignant disease: lessons learned from 46 consecutive procedures. J Am Coll Surg 2003;197(6):902–13.

46. Orringer MB, Marshall B, Iannettoni MD. Transhiatal esophagectomy: clinical experience and refinements. Ann Surg 1999;230(3):392–400 [discussion: 400–3].
47. Luketich JD, Alvelo-Rivera M, Buenaventura PO, et al. Minimally invasive esophagectomy: outcomes in 222 patients. Ann Surg 2003;238(4):486–94 [discussion: 94–5].
48. Braghetto I, Csendes A, Cardemil G, et al. Open transthoracic or transhiatal esophagectomy versus minimally invasive esophagectomy in terms of morbidity, mortality and survival. Surg Endosc 2006;20(11):1681–6.
49. Yim AP, Wan S, Lee TW, et al. VATS lobectomy reduces cytokine responses compared with conventional surgery. Ann Thorac Surg 2000;70(1):243–7.
50. Nagahiro I, Andou A, Aoe M, et al. Pulmonary function, postoperative pain, and serum cytokine level after lobectomy: a comparison of VATS and conventional procedure. Ann Thorac Surg 2001;72(2):362–5.
51. McKenna RJ Jr, Houck WV. New approaches to the minimally invasive treatment of lung cancer. Curr Opin Pulm Med 2005;11(4):282–6.
52. Demmy TL, Curtis JJ. Minimally invasive lobectomy directed toward frail and high-risk patients: a case-control study. Ann Thorac Surg 1999;68(1):194–200.
53. Nakajima J, Takamoto S, Kohno T, et al. Costs of videothoracoscopic surgery versus open resection for patients with of lung carcinoma. Cancer 2000;89(11 Suppl):2497–501.
54. Gress FG, Savides TJ, Sandler A, et al. Endoscopic ultrasonography, fine-needle aspiration biopsy guided by endoscopic ultrasonography, and computed tomography in the preoperative staging of non-small-cell lung cancer: a comparison study. Ann Intern Med 1997;127(8 Pt 1):604–12.
55. Silvestri GA, Hoffman BJ, Bhutani MS, et al. Endoscopic ultrasound with fine-needle aspiration in the diagnosis and staging of lung cancer. Ann Thorac Surg 1996;61(5):1441–5 [discussion: 45–6].
56. Hunerbein M, Ghadimi BM, Haensch W, et al. Transesophageal biopsy of mediastinal and pulmonary tumors by means of endoscopic ultrasound guidance. J Thorac Cardiovasc Surg 1998;116(4):554–9.
57. Silvestri GA, Tanoue LT, Margolis ML, et al. The noninvasive staging of non-small cell lung cancer: the guidelines. Chest 2003;123(1 Suppl):147S–56S.
58. Detterbeck FC, Jantz MA, Wallace M, et al. Invasive mediastinal staging of lung cancer: ACCP evidence-based clinical practice guidelines (2nd edition). Chest 2007;132(3 Suppl):202S–20S.
59. Harewood GC, Wiersema MJ, Edell ES, et al. Cost-minimization analysis of alternative diagnostic approaches in a modeled patient with non-small cell lung cancer and subcarinal lymphadenopathy. Mayo Clin Proc 2002;77(2):155–64.
60. Wallace MB, Silvestri GA, Sahai AV, et al. Endoscopic ultrasound-guided fine needle aspiration for staging patients with carcinoma of the lung. Ann Thorac Surg 2001;72(6):1861–7.
61. Larsen SS, Vilmann P, Krasnik M, et al. Endoscopic ultrasound guided biopsy versus mediastinoscopy for analysis of paratracheal and subcarinal lymph nodes in lung cancer staging. Lung Cancer 2005;48(1):85–92.
62. Vilmann P, Krasnik M, Larsen SS, et al. Transesophageal endoscopic ultrasound-guided fine-needle aspiration (EUS-FNA) and endobronchial ultrasound-guided transbronchial needle aspiration (EBUS-TBNA) biopsy: a combined approach in the evaluation of mediastinal lesions. Endoscopy 2005;37(9):833–9.
63. Wallace MB, Pascual JM, Raimondo M, et al. Minimally invasive endoscopic staging of suspected lung cancer. JAMA 2008;299(5):540–6.
64. Chambers AS, Jordan T, McGranahan T, et al. A new management approach for esophageal perforation. J Thorac Cardiovasc Surg 2005;130(5):1470–1.

65. Wu JT, Mattox KL, Wall MJ Jr. Esophageal perforations: new perspectives and treatment paradigms. J Trauma 2007;63(5):1173–84.
66. Kanshin NN, Pogodina AN. [Transesophageal drainage of the mediastinum in perforating mediastinitis] [in Greek]. Vestn Khir Im I I Grek 1983;130(2):24–7.
67. Abe N, Sugiyama M, Hashimoto Y, et al. Endoscopic nasomediastinal drainage followed by clip application for treatment of delayed esophageal perforation with mediastinitis. Gastrointest Endosc 2001;54(5):646–8.
68. Kahaleh M, Yoshida C, Kane L, et al. EUS drainage of a mediastinal abscess. Gastrointest Endosc 2004;60(1):158–60.
69. Kahaleh M, Shami VM, Conaway MR, et al. Endoscopic ultrasound drainage of pancreatic pseudocyst: a prospective comparison with conventional endoscopic drainage. Endoscopy 2006;38(4):355–9.
70. Chak A, McGee MF, Faulx A, et al. EUS guided natural orifice transvisceral endoscopic surgical (NOTES) approach to the retroperitoneum [abstract]. Gastrointest Endosc 2006;63:AB264.
71. Fritscher-Ravens A, Swain P. Future therapeutic indications for endoscopic ultrasound. Gastrointest Endosc Clin N Am 2005;15(1):189–208, xi.
72. Fritscher-Ravens A, Mosse CA, Mukherjee D, et al. Transluminal endosurgery: single lumen access anastomotic device for flexible endoscopy. Gastrointest Endosc 2003;58(4):585–91.
73. Fritscher-Ravens A, Mosse CA, Ikeda K, et al. Endoscopic transgastric lymphadenectomy by using EUS for selection and guidance. Gastrointest Endosc 2006;63(2):302–6.
74. Fritscher-Ravens A, Mosse CA, Mukherjee D, et al. Transgastric gastropexy and hiatal hernia repair for GERD under EUS control: a porcine model. Gastrointest Endosc 2004;59(1):89–95.
75. Elmunzer BJ, Schomisch SJ, Trunzo JA, et al. EUS in localizing safe alternate access sites for natural orifice transluminal endoscopic surgery: initial experience in a porcine model. Gastrointest Endosc 2009;69(1):108–14.
76. Woodward T, McCluskey D 3rd, Wallace MB, et al. Pilot study of transesophageal endoscopic surgery: NOTES esophagomyotomy, vagotomy, lymphadenectomy. J Laparoendosc Adv Surg Tech A 2008;18(5):743–5.
77. Bergstrom M, Ikeda K, Swain P, et al. Transgastric anastomosis by using flexible endoscopy in a porcine model (with video). Gastrointest Endosc 2006;63(2):307–12.
78. Jagannath SB, Kantsevoy SV, Vaughn CA, et al. Peroral transgastric endoscopic ligation of fallopian tubes with long-term survival in a porcine model. Gastrointest Endosc 2005;61(3):449–53.
79. Park PO, Bergstrom M, Ikeda K, et al. Experimental studies of transgastric gallbladder surgery: cholecystectomy and cholecystogastric anastomosis (videos). Gastrointest Endosc 2005;61(4):601–6.
80. Sumiyama K, Gostout CJ, Rajan E, et al. Transesophageal mediastinoscopy by submucosal endoscopy with mucosal flap safety valve technique. Gastrointest Endosc 2007;65(4):679–83.
81. Gee DW, Willingham FF, Lauwers GY, et al. Natural orifice transesophageal mediastinoscopy and thoracoscopy: a survival series in swine. Surg Endosc 2008; 22(10):2117–22.
82. Fritscher-Ravens A, Patel K, Ghanbari A, et al. Natural orifice transluminal endoscopic surgery (NOTES) in the mediastinum: long-term survival animal experiments in transesophageal access, including minor surgical procedures. Endoscopy 2007;39(10):870–5.

83. Fischer A, Thomusch O, Benz S, et al. Nonoperative treatment of 15 benign esophageal perforations with self-expandable covered metal stents. Ann Thorac Surg 2006;81(2):467–72.
84. Fritscher-Ravens A, Ghanbari A, Cuming T, et al. Comparative study of NOTES alone vs. EUS-guided NOTES procedures. Endoscopy 2008;40(11):925–30.
85. Willingham FF, Gee DW, Lauwers GY, et al. Natural orifice transesophageal mediastinoscopy and thoracoscopy. Surg Endosc 2008;22(4):1042–7.
86. Sumiyama K, Gostout CJ, Rajan E, et al. Pilot study of transesophageal endoscopic epicardial coagulation by submucosal endoscopy with the mucosal flap safety valve technique (with videos). Gastrointest Endosc 2008;67(3):497–501.
87. Mango P, Mas M, Rivera Y, et al. NOTES is successful for vertebral spinal interventions with significant advantages for anterior spinal procedures. Gastrointest Endosc 2008;67(5):AB114.
88. Pasricha PJ, Hawari R, Ahmed I, et al. Submucosal endoscopic esophageal myotomy: a novel experimental approach for the treatment of achalsia. Gastrointest Endosc 2007;65(5):AB92.
89. Woodward T, Bowers S, Asbun H, et al. NOTES in minimally invasive surgical esophagectomy: technique of endoscopic transesophageal mobilization of the esophagus in an animal model, a preliminary study. Gastrointest Endosc 2009; 69(5):AB164.
90. Sumiyama K, Gostout CJ, Rajan E, et al. Pilot study of the porcine uterine horn as an in vivo appendicitis model for development of endoscopic transgastric appendectomy. Gastrointest Endosc 2006;64(5):808–12.
91. Rattner D, Kalloo A. ASGE/SAGES Working Group on Natural Orifice Translumenal Endoscopic Surgery. October 2005. Surg Endosc 2006;20(2):329–33.
92. Richards WO, Rattner DW. Endoluminal and transluminal surgery: no longer if, but when. Surg Endosc 2005;19(4):461–3.
93. Soper NJ. Natural orifice surgery - the next "big thing"? ACS surgery: principles & practice. New York: WebMD Inc; 2005.
94. Perretta S, Allemann P, Dallemagne B, et al. Natural orifice transluminal endoscopic surgery (N.O.T.E.S.) for neoplasia of the chest and mediastinum. Surg Oncol 2009;18(2):177–80.

New Developments in Esophageal Surgery

C. Daniel Smith, MD

KEYWORDS

- Esophagus • Surgery • Minimally invasive surgery
- Gastroesophageal reflux • Esophagectomy • Hiatal hernia
- Laparoscopy • fundoplication

The past decade has seen a convergence of therapeutic endoscopy and gastrointestinal (GI) surgery starting with the joint interest and development of endoscopic antireflux procedures, and most recently with the combined development of Natural Orifice Transluminal Endoscopic Surgery (NOTES). In fact, the development of NOTES has been through a tangible collaboration through NOSCAR (Natural Orifice Surgery Consortium for Assessment and Research), a collaborative venture between the American Society for Gastrointestinal Endoscopy (ASGE) and the Society of American Gastrointestinal and Endoscopic Surgeons (SAGES). NOSCAR typifies the direction that we are headed with regard to interventional management of GI diseases, and especially the esophagus. Rather than simply add a surgeon's perspective to the topics already covered in this publication, this article will cover some new areas of development in esophageal surgery. Specific topics include reviews of long-term outcomes after laparoscopic antireflux surgery, the use of surgically placed implantable device for lower esophageal sphincter (LES) augmentation (Linx), the use of mesh for hiatal hernioplasty, and prone and nonthoracic approaches to minimally invasive esophagectomy (MIE).

LONG-TERM OUTCOMES OF LAPAROSCOPIC ANTIREFLUX SURGERY

Through most of the 1990s, laparoscopic antireflux surgery promised to cure gastroesophageal reflux disease (GERD) and replace proton pump inhibitors (PPIs). Some who felt that the increasing use of PPIs was actually inducing Barrett's esophagus and the more recent increased prevalence of esophageal adenocarcinoma claimed victory over both GERD and the indiscriminant use of PPIs. In 2001, Spechler and colleagues[1] published a 10-year follow-up to their 1992 prospective randomized comparison of surgery versus medical management of GERD. This 1992 study concluded that surgery was more effective than H2 receptor antagonists at controlling GERD.[2] However, this long-term follow-up study declared surgery a failure and even implied that surgery was dangerous. This was based on a statistically nonsignificant finding that more patients in the surgery group had died during the follow-up period.

Department of Surgery, Mayo Clinic Florida, 4500 San Pablo Road, Jacksonville, FL 32224, USA
E-mail address: smith.c.daniel@mayo.edu

Gastrointest Endoscopy Clin N Am 20 (2010) 139–145
doi:10.1016/j.giec.2009.08.003
1052-5157/09/$ – see front matter © 2010 Published by Elsevier Inc.

giendo.theclinics.com

This study induced a significant decline in confidence in antireflux surgery and therefore a decline in the number of patients offered antireflux surgery by their health care providers. Concurrent with this was the realization that laparoscopic antireflux surgery was quite different from open antireflux procedures, if for no other reason than that the skills needed to perform a well-done fundoplication were special and not easily translated by those surgeons comfortable doing other laparoscopic procedures such as cholecystectomy. With this, anecdotal outcomes with laparoscopic fundoplication included mixed results such as high numbers of patients needing to resume antisecretory medications for symptom control, and high rates of redo fundoplication. This further indicted antireflux surgery as ineffective, at times requiring more surgery to manage poor outcomes and complications. The result of this has been most patients with GERD not being offered surgery unless they have more advanced and complicated problems like large hiatal hernia, Barrett's esophagus, or refractory esophagitis.

Over the past 2 to 3 years there have been multiple publications detailing long-term (>10-year) outcomes with laparoscopic antireflux surgery.[3–7] Several of these are summarized in **Table 1**. In summary, it is clear that in centers with extensive experience with the surgical management of GERD, outcomes are excellent with 85% to 90% of patients being highly satisfied with their outcome with good to excellent control of their GERD symptoms. Around 20% to 30% of patients continue to use their antisecretory medication although often for unknown reasons that may not be directly attributable to GERD. In very few patients was surgery a failure as defined by a poor outcome or the need for more surgery. From these studies and our own experience with thousands of patients undergoing antireflux surgery, expertise in not only surgical skill, but also patient selection and a thorough understanding of GERD is necessary to achieve these outcomes. Antireflux surgery is very effective and best provided through centers of excellence where such expertise exists. Patients should not be denied the option of antireflux surgery, but instead, should be guided to those centers where good outcomes have been achieved. This will be increasingly important as patients find themselves with health insurance that will not cover prescription PPIs and will be seeking alternatives to medication, including antireflux surgery.

Table 1
Long-term outcomes of antireflux surgery

Author	No. pts	Follow-up, y	Results
Teixeira 2009 (qol)	143	5.4 (2–11)	92.3% very good or good result 13% using antisecretory meds
Kornmo 2008 (sc)	33	9.75	93% very good or good 52% with gas bloat 3% using antisecretories
Zaninotto 2007 (sc)	145	8.1	86% success 21% using PPIs 9% required redo
Morgenthal 2007 (sc)	166	11.1 (6–13)	93.3% success 30% using PPIs (unknown reasons)
Kelly 2007 (sc)	226	10–14	84% good to excellent 21% using PPIs 17% required redo

Abbreviations: PPI, proton pump inhibitor; pts, patients; qol, quality of life study; sc, symptom control.

LOWER ESOPHAGEAL SPHINCTER AUGMENTATION (LINX)

Over the years there have been several attempts to develop new techniques for augmenting the LES that would avoid the variable outcomes seen with esophagogastric fundoplication (see preceding section). Most have involved endoscopic approaches ranging from suturing to plicate the LES internally (Endocinch) to polymer injection to change the compliance of the LES (Enteryx). Of these recent new techniques, an endoscopic esophagogastric plication (Esophyx) remains the only new technique currently approved by the Food and Drug Administration (FDA). All others (Endocinch, Stretta, Enteryx, Gatekeeper, NDO) either failed to provide a safe or effective treatment, or were unable to establish a sustainable business model. Again, nearly all of these techniques sought to either reproduce a fundoplication or anatomically alter the LES.

The newest venture into developing an effective antireflux barrier between the stomach and esophagus seeks to mechanically reproduce the function of the LES. This implantable device (Linx) is a string of magnetic beads (**Fig. 1**) that is affixed around the distal esophagus at the gastroesophageal junction (**Fig. 2**).[8] Each of the beads in this bracelet carries a weak magnetic force holding the beads opposed, similar to the constricted LES. The force typical of the esophageal body pressure generated with a swallow is enough to disrupt the magnetic force holding these beads together, thereby opening the ring of magnets allowing a swallowed bolus to pass, similar to the relaxation of the LES. Immediately following this bolus passage, the beads reoppose and the distal esophagus is again closed. This device is placed laparoscopically in a manner similar to how a laparoscopic fundoplication is performed. In contrast to a fundoplication, there is very little dissection and manipulation of the gastric fundus necessary, and the result is very reproducible and predictable. This device is currently only available through an FDA trial.

A feasibility study involved 38 patients who underwent implant of the device over a 1-year period.[9] No intraoperative complications occurred and all patients were

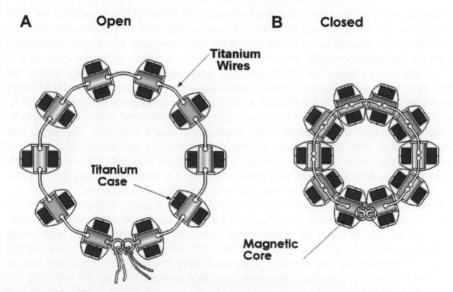

Fig. 1. Bracelet of magnetic beads depicting (*A*) the magnetic force between the beads broken and the beads distracted and ring open, and (*B*) the magnetic force between the beads intake and the ring closed. (*From* Ganz RA, Gostout CJ, Grudem J, et al. Use of a magnetic sphincter for the treatment of GERD: a feasibility study. Gastrointest Endosc 2008;67(2):287–94.)

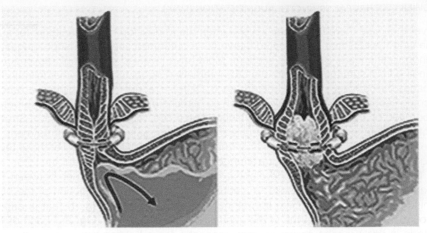

Fig. 2. Illustration of the placement and function of the Linx device.

discharged from the hospital within 48 hours. At an average follow-up of 7 months (12–434 days) the GERD-Health Related Quality of Life (HRQL) was significantly decreased (26.0 to 1.0, $P<.005$). At 3 months postoperatively, 79% had normalized their 24-hour pH test and 89% were off of all antireflux medication. All patients could belch and no migrations or erosions had occurred. This device promises an easy, reproducible procedure where the native function of the LES can be augmented. Preliminarily it appears to be one of those simple inventions that may prove to be one of the most successful.

THE USE OF MESH FOR HIATAL HERNIOPLASTY

One of the most vexing anatomic defects associated with GERD is a hiatal hernia. With a hiatal hernia the LES loses its anatomic association with the diaphragm, thereby diminishing the augmentation of the LES from the diaphragm. It is a well-established principle that when surgically correcting GERD with a fundoplication, it is important to return the LES to below the diaphragm and repair any associated hiatal defect. By definition, those who develop a hiatal hernia have an underlying propensity to hiatal hernia formation, either in the form of weak tissue comprising the esophageal hiatus, obesity, or both. Advanced age is strongly associated with hiatal hernia, supporting an underlying etiology of weakening of the esophageal hiatus over time. Therefore, one could assume that simple repair of the defect without somehow reinforcing or enhancing the repair will likely eventually break down and fail. This has certainly been the case with abdominal wall hernias, where it is well established that the use of mesh in the repair of these hernias leads to low rates of recurrence.

Despite the acceptance of the use of mesh in repair of abdominal wall hernias, the use of mesh in hiatal hernia repair has not gained acceptance until recently. Proponents of the use of mesh for hiatal hernia repair invoke the abdominal wall hernia data along with the high recurrent hernia rate with suture-only repair of hiatal hernias as the justification for use of mesh. They also point out that newer meshes induce a more blunted inflammatory response, and that new techniques for isolating the mesh from the vicinity of the esophagus should prevent esophageal contact and ultimate erosion.[10]

Opponents of the use of mesh for hiatal hernia repair have strongly pointed out that the diaphragm is not the same as the skeletal muscle of the abdominal wall. The region of the esophageal hiatus is extremely dynamic making any prosthetic that induces scarring and the associated stiffness problematic. The presence of an artificial material next to the esophagus that induces scarring and inflammation is destined to cause esophageal inflammation, ulceration, and eventual erosion. In fact, there have been several case reports of mesh placed at the esophageal hiatus causing esophageal erosion and the eventual need for esophagectomy.[11] Most recently, absorbable meshes have been developed and used for hiatal hernia repair. The idea that the mesh eventually dissolves thereby avoiding any long-term impact on the diaphragm and esophagus is appealing. A prospective randomized trial of a biologic mesh versus no mesh at all showed a statistically significant reduction in the recurrence rate at 6 months postoperatively.[12] Twenty-four percent of patients undergoing hiatal hernia repair without mesh developed a recurrent hernia 6 months after surgery in comparison with 9% of patients who underwent repair with the absorbable mesh. Although the patients who underwent mesh hernia repair had more dysphagia than those without mesh placed, all patients had their dysphagia resolve without specific intervention. No patients experienced a significant complication of mesh placement. The authors conclude that an absorbable mesh reduces recurrence and should be used routinely for hiatal hernia repair. No long-term data are available to support that the benefit of the mesh is durable after it has been completely absorbed. These data suggest, however, that mesh may have a role in hiatal hernia repair. Because the consequence of a complication related to the mesh such as erosion or stricture may require esophagectomy, cautious and limited use of mesh is still recommended. Additionally, a recurrent hiatal hernia is often not clinically significant with only a small percentage of patients with a recurrence actually having significant symptoms.[13]

MINIMALLY INVASIVE ESOPHAGECTOMY, PRONE AND NONTHORACIC APPROACHES

Minimally invasive esophagectomy (MIE) uses laparoscopy and thoracoscopy to perform procedures comparable to transhiatal or Ivor Lewis esophagectomy. Whether a two-field (abdomen and chest) or three-field (abdomen, chest and neck) approach, MIE typically uses right lateral decubitus positioning for thoracoscopic esophageal mobilization followed by laparoscopy with cervical anastomosis. The lateral decubitus position provides access to the chest from a vantage point comparable to open thoracotomy. Because the esophagus is a medial and posterior structure, to gain exposure and access to the esophagus through this approach, four to five trocars are needed along with a skilled assistant to provide adequate exposure. Often an enlarged incision is needed to allow the insertion of instruments needed for exposure and to keep the operative field free of blood.

Recently, the prone approach to thoracic access for esophagectomy has been developed (**Fig. 3**).[14–16] This approach takes advantage of the medial and posterior location of the esophagus by allowing the lung and mediastinal structures to fall away from the esophagus without any additional retraction beyond the exposure provided from gravity alone. This position also allows any blood that might accumulate to fall away from the operative field providing a clear view without additional maneuvers. When the prone approach is used, frequently only three trocars are necessary, thereby minimizing the morbidity of the additional points of access. Using this technique, several investigators have been able to demonstrate shorter operative times, less blood loss, decreased length of stay, and adequate resection margins and lymphadenectomy. This technique promises to further evolve MIE providing patients with incremental outcome benefits from not only an open esophagectomy, but also from the currently most common lateral approach MIE.

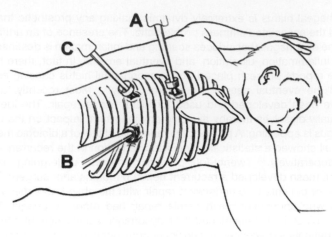

Fig. 3. Patient positioning and trocar placement for prone minimally invasive esophagectomy (MIE).

Finally, under development is a nonthoracic cage approach to esophageal mobilization. With this technique, the neck incision used for proximal esophageal isolation and eventual esophagogastrotomy is used to gain access to the mediastinum and chest to mobilize the esophagus. This technique is an extension of some of the techniques used in NOTES and single incision laparoscopic surgery. In each of these techniques, advanced in-line instrumentation allows visualization and tissue manipulation, thereby allowing access through a single small point of access. During esophagectomy, the placement of a port through the neck incision and across the thoracic inlet into the chest allows full access to the intrathoracic esophagus to perform a visualized dissection and mobilization. Preliminary work confirms that with this technique, no incisions through the chest wall are necessary to achieve the same result as when the chest wall is breached. This technique would essentially eliminate the morbidity of the chest incisions and further enhance recovery and limit complications.

In summary, recent advances in esophageal surgery are confirming the role of antireflux surgery in the management of GERD, development of an LES augmentation device for GERD, clarifying the potential role of mesh use in the repair of hiatal hernias, and refining techniques in minimally invasive esophagectomy, thereby reducing the morbidity of this important potentially curative approach to early esophageal cancer.

REFERENCES

1. Spechler SJ, Lee E, Ahnen D, et al. Long-term outcome of medical and surgical therapies for gastroesophageal reflux disease: follow-up of a randomized controlled trial [see comment]. JAMA 2001;285(18):2331–8.
2. Spechler SJ. Comparison of medical and surgical therapy for complicated gastroesophageal reflux disease in veterans. The Department of Veterans Affairs Gastroesophageal Reflux Disease Study Group [see comment]. N Engl J Med 1992;326(12):786–92.
3. Teixeira JP, Mosquera V, Flores A. Long-term outcomes of quality of life after laparoscopic Nissen fundoplication. Hepatogastroenterology 2009;56(89):80–4.
4. Kornmo TS, Ruud TE. Long-term results of laparoscopic Nissen fundoplication due to gastroesophageal reflux disease. A ten year follow-up in a low volume center. Scand J Surg 2008;97(3):227–30.

5. Zaninotto G, Portale G, Costantini M, et al. Long-term results (6–10 years) of laparoscopic fundoplication. J Gastrointest Surg 2007;11(9):1138–45.
6. Morgenthal CB, Shane MD, Stival A, et al. The durability of laparoscopic Nissen fundoplication: 11-year outcomes [see comment]. J Gastrointest Surg 2007;11(6): 693–700.
7. Kelly JJ, Watson DI, Chin KF, et al. Laparoscopic Nissen fundoplication: clinical outcomes at 10 years. J Am Coll Surg 2007;205(4):570–5.
8. Ganz RA, Gostout CJ, Grudem J, et al. Use of a magnetic sphincter for the treatment of GERD: a feasibility study [see comment]. Gastrointest Endosc 2008; 67(2):287–94.
9. Bonavina L, Saino GI, Bona D, et al. Magnetic augmentation of the lower esophageal sphincter: results of a feasibility clinical trial. J Gastrointest Surg 2008; 12(12):2133–40.
10. Johnson JM, Carbonell AM, Carmody BJ, et al. Laparoscopic mesh hiatoplasty for paraesophageal hernias and fundoplications: a critical analysis of the available literature. Surg Endosc 2006;20(3):362–6.
11. Griffith PS, Valenti V, Qurashi K, et al. Rejection of goretex mesh used in prosthetic cruroplasty: a case series. Int J Surg 2008;6(2):106–9.
12. Oelschlager BK, Pellegrini CA, Hunter J, et al. Biologic prosthesis reduces recurrence after laparoscopic paraesophageal hernia repair: a multicenter, prospective, randomized trial [see comment]. Ann Surg 2006;244(4):481–90.
13. Mattar SG, Bowers SP, Galloway KD, et al. Long-term outcome of laparoscopic repair of paraesophageal hernia. Surg Endosc 2002;16(5):745–9.
14. Dapri G, Himpens J, Cadiere GB. Minimally invasive esophagectomy for cancer: laparoscopic transhiatal procedure or thoracoscopy in prone position followed by laparoscopy? Surg Endosc 2008;22(4):1060–9.
15. Fabian T, McKelvey AA, Kent MS, et al. Prone thoracoscopic esophageal mobilization for minimally invasive esophagectomy. Surg Endosc 2007;21(9):1667–70.
16. Palanivelu C, Prakash A, Senthilkumar R, et al. Minimally invasive esophagectomy: thoracoscopic mobilization of the esophagus and mediastinal lymphadenectomy in prone position–experience of 130 patients. J Am Coll Surg 2006; 203(1):7–16.

The Future of Endoscopic Esophageal Therapy—What Comes Next

Robert A. Ganz, MD, FASGE[a,b,c],*

KEYWORDS

- Esophagus • Endoscopy • Ablation • Reflux
- Barrett's esophagus

"Nanotechnology will change everything."
—*Shimon Peres, President of Israel, in a speech at Technion University, 2008
Haifa, Israel*
"The most important thing in life is not to know where one is but where one is going."
—*Goethe*

If the past is prologue, based on the recent rapid and significant changes in the endoscopic diagnosis and therapy of esophageal diseases over the past several years, one can anticipate continued, accelerating new developments in the field. These new developments will be based on continuing advancements in the basic sciences of optics, physics, cell biology, and nanotechnology, and will transform the clinical practice of esophagology radically, in some ways expanding the diagnostic role of primary care, and in other ways transforming treatment of the esophagus and its disorders into a complex subspecialty within the sphere of gastroenterology.

To begin with, optical technology exists that inevitably will shift initial diagnostic endoscopy to primary care physicians or to midlevel nursing or technical providers. Current endoscopic practice generally requires sedation, nursing assistance, recovery facilities, and scope disinfection. Gastroenterologists perform most endoscopic examinations under white light endoscopy, and are taught to recognize endoscopic abnormalities via repetitive training procedures and examinations. In the near future,

[a] Minnesota Gastroenterology, PA, 5705 West Old Shakopee Road, Suite #150, Bloomington, MN 55437, USA
[b] Department of Medicine, Abbott-Northwestern Hospital, 800 E. 28th Street, Minneapolis, MN 55407, USA
[c] Department of Medicine, University of Minnesota, 500 Harvard Street, Minneapolis, MN 55455, USA
* Minnesota Gastroenterology, PA, 5705 West Old Shakopee Road, Suite #150, Bloomington, MN 55437.
E-mail address: gastrodude@visi.com

Gastrointest Endoscopy Clin N Am 20 (2010) 147–159
doi:10.1016/j.giec.2009.07.010
1052-5157/09/$ – see front matter © 2010 Elsevier Inc. All rights reserved.

giendo.theclinics.com

however, primary care providers will readily be able to perform painless, nonsedated upper endoscopies using either disposable naked endoscopic fibers or reinforced endoscopic catheters that can be passed either transnasally or orally, quickly and comfortably (Third Eye Retroscope technology, Avantis Medical, Sunnyvale, California).[1] Rather than have primary care providers trained in endoscopic recognition, these office-based endoscopic examinations can be transmitted in real time, or can be recorded for later viewing, via fiberoptic or cable transmission technology, and they can be reviewed or read remotely either on portable computers, specified image readers, or cell phones. In the future, it is entirely probable that gastroenterologists will contract out their services to primary care clinics for reviewing or over-reading of initial diagnostic endoscopic examinations. One can imagine a situation whereby an expert gastroenterologist, anywhere in the country, can be called upon, or contracted to review complex endoscopic video or images. This service also could be outsourced and readily performed by expert overseas providers. Because much of foregut endoscopy involves the diagnosis or screening of gastroesophageal reflux disease (GERD)-related disorders, esophageal endoscopic practice will be affected dramatically by this development. It is also not inconceivable that given the development of remote robotics, an expert gastroenterologist can consult and take over the controls of a real-time endoscopic examination remotely in a distant primary care office.

Another competing technology in this arena is the advent of steerable or directional video capsules. Using piezovibrating elements, or using directional magnets, endoscopic video capsules can be directed reliably in the esophagus, stomach and small intestine, and areas of interest can be studied similar to endoscopic examinations.[2] Certainly one can conceive of directional capsule endoscopy being used in primary care offices for initial diagnostic examinations, particularly in the areas of gastroesophageal (GE) reflux and to screen for Barrett's esophagus and esophageal cancer. Nondirectional capsules also can be used for initial diagnostic examinations, although they have not yet achieved the same level of diagnostic accuracy as upper endoscopy. Nonetheless, these studies are significantly less expensive than standard sedated endoscopy. In the future, one can conceive of a patient with upper abdominal dyspepsia or heartburn, being directed by his or her primary care physician to purchase an inexpensive battery-powered video capsule at their local drug store, then swallow the capsule at home, and have the downloaded images transmitted to the primary care clinic or gastroenterology office for later viewing.

GERD—DIAGNOSIS

The endoscopic diagnosis and treatment of GERD will change dramatically in coming years. Current endoscopic assessment of reflux is binary; patients either have nonerosive reflux disease, in which case the diagnosis cannot be confirmed endoscopically, or there is grossly evident erosive disease that is diagnostic, however, relatively uncommon. In the future, however, very precise endoscopic assessments of GE reflux will be developed; in particular one will be able to measure and assess early disruption and increased spacing of esophageal epithelial intracellular tight junctions, which is considered to be the earliest histologic sign of GERD.[3,4] Using confocal endoscopic imaging, assessment of intracellular spacing can be determined with a high degree of reproducibility and corresponds to microscopic histologic samples. With this technology, patients with grossly nonerosive esophageal mucosal findings can be subcategorized into those with early cellular changes consistent with GE reflux, versus those with no confocal microscopic changes.

Using this technology in conjunction with pH profiles, one also could determine response to therapy.[3,4] It would be highly unlikely that patients with restored normal epithelial intracellular spacing would continue to have symptomatic heartburn. Thus patients with ongoing reflux symptoms, and those with functional complaints, should be readily discernible. Antiacid medication also would be titratable to intracellular spacing, and one should be readily able to determine nonerosive GERD patients with true failed medical management.

Another coming advance in the realm of GERD diagnostics is the endoscopic functional luminal imaging procedure or Endo-FLIP (Crospon Diagnostics, Galway, Ireland).[5] The FLIP technology involves placing a deflated volume-based Barostat bag through the biopsy channel of the endoscope, positioning the Barostat bag across the GE junction, and slowly inflating it with water to obtain a high-fidelity measurement of the cross-sectional diameter of this region. As the Barostat bag is filled with water, pressure sensors within the bag construct a three-dimensional image of the GE junction and lower esophageal sphincter (LES). The determined cross-sectional diameter and distensibility of the esophagus in the region of the GE junction is an accurate indicator of lateral displacement of the diaphragmatic crus, and it indirectly measures LES compliance in this area and GE yield pressure.[5] It has become clear in recent years that measurement of the LES pressure (ie, squeeze pressure) is not particularly valuable in predicting GERD, because most GERD patients actually have normal LES pressures.[6]

The FLIP procedure can assess the more important LES compliance or gastric yield (ie, the ability of the GE junction to resist opening from elevated gastric volumes and pressures as patients fill their stomachs with food or air). The compliance of this area or the pressure at which the GE junction yields to increased gastric volumes is likely to be a much more accurate predictor of GERD and is the functional equivalent of the endoscopic Hill grade anatomy assessment.[7] This technique also helps determine lateral displacement of the diaphragmatic crus, which is a key, but previously immeasurable, component of GE reflux. Current endoscopic practice can assess only axial displacement of the GE junction proximal to the diaphragm (ie, a sliding hiatal hernia); however, this is a highly variable and inaccurate measure, particularly as regards reducible, sliding hiatal hernias.

GERD—NEW THERAPEUTIC OPTIONS

Regarding future endoscopic therapy for GERD, there are several exciting developments to anticipate. One potential development is the option of stem cell injection directly into the area of the LES, with biologic regrowth of LES cells and restoration of sphincter dynamics. In recent years, it has become possible to extract human somatic cells and via bacteriophage viral genomic or drug manipulation, convert ordinary somatic cells into inducible pluripotent stem cells.[8] When these inducible pluripotent stem cells are injected into target LES tissue with the proper milieu characteristics, the stem cells can regenerate into LES sphincter cells and restore normal sphincter squeeze characteristics. Success of this technology, however, likely will depend on other reflux parameters including a patient's anatomy, axial displacement of the native LES, lateral displacement of the diaphragmatic crus, and whether the native LES was normal or hypotensive to begin with.

Endoscopic, endoluminal antireflux devices have failed in the past, including

Various sewing and plicating devices (BARD endocinch, Murray Hill, New Jersey; HizWhiz; NDO plicator, Mansfield, Massachusetts)
Radiofrequency devices intended to tighten the LES (Stretta, Curon Inc, Fremont, California)

Injectable devices that either tried to impact sphincter compliance (Enteryx) or narrow the lumen in the region of the LES to create resistance to retrograde flow (Gatekeeper, Medtronic Inc, Fridley, Minnesota)

There are new developments in this area, however. Durasphere (Carbon Medical Technologies, Maple Grove, Minnesota) is a new injectable bulking agent composed of micronized carbon spheres that are injected in the region of the GE junction.[9] A recent pilot publication has demonstrated feasibility of this agent for treating GERD and has shown that the microcarbon spheres are safe, durable, effective and nonmigratory. In this small study, 70% of patients with mild-to-moderate GERD were able to discontinue all reflux medications at 12 months, and 40% normalized their pH scores. Moreover, the technique is simple and caused no postprocedure pain or dysphagia.[9] Another new device (Esophyx, Endogastric Solutions Inc, Redmond, Washington) tries to create an endoscopic Nissen fundoplication in an endoluminal fashion, although results to date have been suboptimal.[10]

The LINX device (Torax Medical Incorporated, Shoreview, Minnesota) is a beaded magnetic bracelet that is placed around the esophagus in the region of the LES. The individual magnetic beads spread apart to allow food to pass, and to provide for belching and vomiting, but then re-attract to restore compliance and yield pressure dynamics at the GE junction.[11,12] Extensive animal testing and early human clinical data with some patients followed out to 3 years have shown this device to be very safe with no reported migration or erosion to date. The device does not appear to affect resting LES tone; rather it appears to prevent inappropriate LES opening. Early clinical data appear impressive for this device; in a recent study of 44 implanted GERD patients, 80% achieved a normal acid pH score at 1 year, and 90% completely eliminated the need for any antiacid medication. GERD health-related quality of life scores improved from initial values of 26.5 to 1 year scores of 3.0.[11,12] The LINX device is placed laparoscopically, and is technically simpler and quicker than performing a Nissen fundoplication. The procedure is being performed on an outpatient basis, and patients can resume standard diets later that day. There is also the possibility for endoscopic placement of the device via a natural orifice transluminal endoscopic approach (NOTES). The device has significant potential in obviating the need for Nissen fundoplication in many severe GERD patients, and it can extend device therapy to the many reflux patients dissatisfied with medical management but not willing to undergo the physiologic disruption of a Nissen procedure.

Given the previous discussion, it is clear that the current practice of GERD will change dramatically in the future. Current practice involves maintaining virtually all GERD patients on proton pump inhibitor therapy, recognizing that a significant percentage of patients will remain dissatisfied, with referral of only a select few severe GERD patients to Nissen surgery. In the future, given some of the just described new diagnostic entities, one will be able to

better and more accurately subcategorize GERD patients into those most amenable to medical, endoscopic, or surgical management

choose the most appropriate therapy for an individual patient based on LES pressure, length, compliance and yield pressure, microscopic intracellular dynamics, lateral displacement of the diaphragmatic crus, axial displacement of the GE junction, and pH characteristics.

The range of therapeutic options also will increase, giving practitioners the ability to tailor specific therapies to specific physiologic deficits, resulting in better outcomes.

EOSINOPHILIC ESOPHAGITIS

Current endoscopic practice for diagnosing eosinophilic esophagitis involves visual inspection, searching for mucosal edema, multiple rings or mucosal furrowing, and evidence of luminal narrowing or stricture formation. Random endoscopic biopsies also are obtained looking for eosinophilic infiltration in the esophageal mucosa.[13] Unfortunately, current endoscopic diagnosis of eosinophilic esophagitis is problematic, however, because of the fact that approximately 30% of patients with eosinophilic esophagitis have normal-appearing mucosa. Additionally, the disease is often patchy, requiring numerous random biopsies over several regions of the esophagus. Moreover, the exact density of eosinophils per high-powered field has not been established for accurate diagnosis. A count of 15 intraepithelial eosinophils per high-powered field is considered to be the absolute minimum number to make a diagnosis in the context of accompanying symptoms and endoscopic findings, but the methods for enumerating eosinophils is highly variable, and there is not consensus on this issue.[14] Furthermore, using this minimum number, a single biopsy specimen only has an approximate 55% sensitivity in the diagnosis of eosinophilic esophagitis, whereas five or more specimens have a sensitivity approaching 100%.[15] Treatment of this disease is also problematic. Elimination diets often are recommended under the supervision of a registered dietitian, but even when this approach is successful, it is unclear which food group is actually responsible for the eosinophilic infiltration, and it is difficult to determine which food groups can be reintroduced with safety. Topical or systemic corticosteroids also may be used, with oral fluticasone as the preferred agent; however, in a recent double-blind, placebo-controlled trial, only 50% of patients with eosinophilic esophagitis responded to this therapy.[16]

It would be ideal to have an endoscopic technology that could readily and more accurately measure and grade eosinophilic infiltration of the esophagus compared with biopsy and histology, and rapidly assess response to specific food group avoidances. In the future, rather than assess gross endoscopic visual findings and histology, practitioners may be using technology similar to Endo-FLIP to rapidly and accurately determine esophageal wall compliance. Esophageal wall compliance should correlate to the degree of eosinophilic infiltration, and practitioners may be able to more accurately characterize the degree of disease via serial compliance measurements in the body of the esophagus. Future patients with presumed eosinophilic esophagitis could have a baseline FLIP measurement obtained, confirming the diagnosis. Patients then would be entered into an elimination diet protocol, with a repeat FLIP examination used to document improvement. The reintroduction of specific foods with serial compliance measurements then could determine rapidly which specific food group needs to be avoided. This new way of measuring and assessing esophageal wall compliance could obviate the need for steroid use and might eliminate discrepancies based on random biopsy and interobserver disagreement of density of histologic eosinophilic infiltration.[5]

BARRETT'S ESOPHAGUS—DIAGNOSIS AND RISK STRATIFICATION

Adenocarcinoma of the esophagus and gastric cardia is the most rapidly rising cancer in the United States and Western Europe today; at present rates of rise, a decade from now one can anticipate over 40,000 cancers of the esophagus annually in the United States.[17] The proximate cause of adenocarcinoma of the esophagus is the epidemic of GERD and consequent Barrett's esophagus, but current endoscopic technology limits the ability to screen for Barrett's esophagus and the ability to determine those at risk for progression versus those with stable disease. As noted in the previous discussion, technological advancements likely will allow mass screening via primary care, although the cost-effectiveness of this approach remains to be determined.

Rapid advances in cellular genetics and microarray technology should help practitioners better stratify patients at risk of progressing to dysplasia and cancer, and help better target therapy.[18] Microarray technology evolved from Southern blotting, where fragmented DNA was attached to various substrates and then probed with a known gene or fragment. Current DNA or RNA multiplex microarray technology consists of arrayed series of thousands, or even tens of thousands, of microscopic spots of genetic oligonucleotides, each containing specific DNA or RNA sequences such as a gene chip, or Affymetrix chip (Affymetric Inc, Santa Clara, California). These arrays can be used to detect single nucleotide polymorphisms (SNPs) among alleles in a specific patient or within populations, assessing predisposition to disease. These microarrays also can be used to measure gene expression levels in a technique known as DNA expression analysis or expression profiling.

The promise of these powerful genetic amplification techniques would be the ability to accurately predict

Which GERD patients (or even non-GERD patients) would have the genetic basis to potentially progress to Barrett's esophagus

Which Barrett's esophagus patients would be at genetic risk to progress to dysplasia or cancer

Of those at highest risk to progress, which patients would respond best to ablative therapies.

The genetic techniques also should prove helpful in risk-stratifying siblings with or without baseline reflux disease.[18]

Advances in optical imaging technology also will enhance greatly future ability to survey those diagnosed with Barrett's esophagus and hopefully will allow for more accurate stratification of patients into various risk categories. It is known that existing histologic light microscopy techniques in the pathology laboratory are problematic in distinguishing metaplastic Barrett's esophagus from dysplastic Barrett's esophagus. Moreover, interobserver pathologic agreement for both low-grade dysplasia and high-grade dysplasia is poor, with multiple studies demonstrating an inability to obtain histologic consensus. Expert pathologic agreement for the diagnosis of low-grade dysplasia is only around 30%, and agreement for high-grade dysplasia is approximately 60%. Thus the field is ripe for optical imaging improvements that will inform better decision making in Barrett's esophagus.[19]

In fact, there are numerous exciting, new optical technologies competing in this arena. Narrow band imaging (NBI) is an optical advance that enhances mucosal surface detail without the need for chromoendoscopy, which previously required dyes or contrast stains. In standard white light endoscopy, all of the visible light spectra illuminate the mucosa, including colors with relatively short wavelengths (blue–green) and colors with longer wavelengths (red) and deeper penetration into tissue. In narrow band imaging, the light is filtered, allowing only the shorter wavelengths to illuminate the mucosa, resulting in opacification of the deeper layers and preferential surface enhancement of the mucosa. This allows for more accurate characterization of mucosal cells and has been proven to be useful in detecting Barrett's esophagus and Barrett's dysplasia. In a recent study of 30 patients with Barrett's esophagus involving almost 200 biopsy specimens, various structural patterns of Barrett's mucosa could be identified, including a tubular/villous pattern, a circular pattern, and a distorted or irregular pattern with a high degree of accuracy. Barrett's esophagus containing high-grade dysplasia also could be recognized with sensitivity, specificity, and positive predictive values approaching 100%. Most characteristic of high-grade dysplasia were areas of irregularity in the surface mucosa associated with abnormal and tortuous capillary vessels.[20] Another prospective, blinded, tandem endoscopy study from Mayo Clinic, Rochester, Minnesota, compared NBI with standard endoscopy in patients with Barrett's esophagus. Higher grades of dysplasia were found by NBI, and NBI-directed biopsies detected dysplasia in more patients. Moreover, NBI required fewer biopsy samples compared with standard white light endoscopy.[21]

Confocal endomicroscopy is a fusion of endoscopy and confocal microscopic imaging. To create precise confocal images, blue laser light is focused on the desired tissue. Topically applied fluorescent materials (typically fluorescein sodium), are excited by the laser light, and the confocal optical unit exclusively detects the fluorescing light in an exactly defined horizontal plane. This technology allows confocal images via an endoscope, yielding 1000 times magnification, a 0.7 μ limit of resolution, and subsurface depth penetration of 250 μ, allowing high-resolution assessment of epithelial cells and cellular nuclei, and also allowing for optical sectioning deeper into the mucosa including identification of histologic features of lamina propria, blood vessels, basement membrane integrity, connective tissue, and inflammatory cells.

Recent studies have determined that use of confocal endomicroscopy is feasible in endoscopy, with a high degree of accuracy in diagnosing Barrett's esophagus and in distinguishing metaplastic from dysplastic Barrett's epithelium. In a recent study involving 63 patients with Barrett's esophagus, digital confocal images were compared with standard histopathology. In this trial, Barrett's esophagus and associated neoplasia were predicted with a sensitivity of 98.1% and 92.9%, and a specificity of 94.1%, and 98.4%, respectively.[22]

An even more exciting application of confocal endomicroscopy, however, is in conjunction with fluorescent probes. The gene coding for fluorescence in jellyfish was identified recently, and it can be incorporated into cells for rapid endoscopic identification. This fluorescence characteristic can be incorporated into probe peptides for rapid identification of early dysplastic tissue. Phage libraries of small peptide probes can identify sequences of dysplasia anywhere in the gastrointestinal (GI) tract, including the colon, but in particular, they can be constructed for Barrett's esophagus. These fluorescein-conjugated heptapeptides can be used as targeting probes for early identification of dysplasia or for early cancer detection. Previous attempts at fluorescence binding using small molecules, antibodies, and antibody fragments met with only limited success, because the these probes were relatively large, had slow binding kinetics, and did not penetrate into diseased tissues very well. Peptides, however, are small, bind rapidly, and penetrate into epithelium easily and quickly. The peptides are analogous to painting a wall; basically they are sprayed on, or swallowed by the patient, penetrate and bind to dysplastic tissue, and are able to be imaged within a few minutes.[23]

Once bound, the fluorescence signal within the peptide can readily be identified by confocal imaging with the area of abnormality localized. This technique can pick up even a single dysplastic cell with a high degree of accuracy, in vivo, in real time. Once these abnormal areas are imaged, they can then be readily treated endoscopically using various resection or ablative techniques. It is quite likely that in the future combinations of peptides may be required, and confocal imaging techniques with much broader endoscopic views would be clinically useful. These latter techniques are in development.

At some point in the future it also may be possible to implant a sort of fluorescence tattoo on the epithelium of patients with Barrett's esophagus that would change color if neoplastic alterations occurred.[23]

Optical coherence tomography (OCT) is optically analogous to sound waves that employ high-frequency ultrasound, which either passes through or bounces off of tissue. Using the technique of low coherence light interferometry background light scattering is measured as the light passes through various tissues and cellular structures, and the intensity of the light scatter can be measured and reconstructed as high-resolution images in vivo and in real time. OCT devices currently in clinical use are probe-based, passing through endoscope channels, and they can be used in either a linear or radial scanning fashion. These devices typically supply a sampling depth of approximately 1 to 2 mm and a tissue resolution of roughly 10 μ, although probes in current development will be able to obtain resolutions as low as 2 to 5 μ. Studies using OCT probes in patients with Barrett's esophagus have been promising; however, further refinement of this technique is required. In one study evaluating approximately 200 OCT images matched with biopsy-acquired histology, sensitivity and specificity for diagnosing Barrett's high-grade dysplasia and intramucosal carcinoma were 75% and 83%, respectively.[24]

An exciting new development in the realm of OCT involves marrying this technique with infrared spectroscopy in a technique called angle-resolved low coherence interferometry. Similar to OCT, light scattering is measured; however, in this technique, light is measured as a function of the scattering angle, and computational models invert the angles and deduce the size of the scattering tissue elements.[25] The main advantage of the combined technique is the ability to accurately assess mucosal structures at varying depths. This technique has shown great promise in measuring the average size of cell nuclei. A recent presentation of this technique involving an experimental animal model of Barrett's esophagus distinguished normal and dysplastic epithelium with a high degree of sensitivity and specificity. This technique also has the promise of wide-field scanning and potentially could be used as a red-flag technique in surveying Barrett's esophagus.[25]

There are several other spectroscopic techniques being assessed, including fluorescent spectroscopy, elastic scattering spectroscopy, and Raman spectroscopy. These modalities all involve measuring light tissue scattering interactions, to obtain tissue architectural and cellular and subcellular component information. Light of varying wavelengths and intensities can be fired to stimulate and interact with tissue; this interaction of stimulation and scattering yields distinct optical fingerprints that then can be correlated and analyzed to reconstruct images.[26]

Fluorescence spectrophotometry takes advantage of natural, endogenous tissue fluorophores that can be stimulated by light, or the tissue can be enhanced by the topical or exogenous administration of fluorophores such as those used in photodynamic therapy (eg, hematoporphyrin and aminolevulinic acid). As tissue progresses from metaplasia to dysplasia, alterations in tissue characteristics will cause fluorescing light to bounce off in different, specific, and recognizable patterns.

Autofluorescence endoscopy is an extension of this technique that excites endogenous tissue fluorophores via light emitted from an endoscope, in real time, based on varying ratios of blue, red, and green light. Light is stimulated by various sources (eg, xenon lamp) and separated and fractionated by rotary filters. Dysplastic tissue containing altered fluorophore content displays a relatively longer wavelength and a different color compared with normal, nondysplastic tissue. Using initial endoscopic autofluorescence designs, a variety of results have been reported for detecting dysplasia in the esophagus. A digital high-resolution system recently was introduced that appears more promising in differentiating dysplastic and neoplastic lesions.[27]

Raman spectroscopy is a technique that detects laser-stimulated scattered light that has undergone alterations in wavelength. Raman detected light can be very detailed and can assess tissue vibration down to the level of molecular bonds. As such, Raman spectroscopy has great potential for detailed diagnosis; however, the signals are weak and require augmentation equipment that is currently not suitable for attachment or mounting on an endoscope.

Perhaps the most promising of all the spectroscopic techniques is elastic light scattering spectroscopy (ELSS). This technique does not involve changes in wavelength; rather an algorithm measures light scatter as it interacts with various tissues. The amount of scattered light has been shown to closely correlate with nuclear size and density, and thus it is a predictor of dysplasia. Initial studies of reflectance spectroscopy in Barrett's esophagus have shown good sensitivities and specificities in the detection of dysplasia. This technique also has been shown to correlate with various cell constituents such as collagen and hemoglobin. Some tissue components, such as collagen, scatter light, and other components, such as hemoglobin, absorb light.

By taking advantage of this varying light scatter and absorption, a recently reported modification of ELSS, called four-dimensional elastic light-scattering fingerprinting (4D-ELF), allows for detection of microvascular blood content and thus can be used as a field effect technique for assessing early dysplastic changes. This technique recently was reported to assess early angiogenesis in colon carcinogenesis, and it can distinguish normal colonic mucosa from microvascular blood flow in patients with both small and large polyps. As patients form adenomatous polyps, there is an early microvascular increase in blood supply because of the neoplastic (albeit benign) nature of the polyp tissue. This effect can be detected regionally, adjacent to the polyp, but in a stunning application, this effect also can be detected throughout the colon, even if the polyp is in a remote location.[28]

In other words, a polyp anywhere in the colon will cause an increase in microvascular blood supply throughout the entire organ, and this effect can be picked up by the 4D-ELF technique. Thus probing the rectum can detect polyps in the right colon or cecum. The microvascular signal increases in intensity as the polyp is neared, sort of like a divining stick, and it can be used to localize hidden polyps. As polyps enlarge and then progress to cancer, the microvascular blood supply increases, and this change can be detected as well, allowing the technique to distinguish normal colon, from small polyp to large polyp to cancer.[28] This breakthrough technology will be able to be applied to the esophagus also, because normal esophageal mucosa, Barrett's metaplasia, Barrett's low-grade dysplasia, high-grade dysplasia, and adenocarcinoma the esophagus all should induce recognizable differences in microvascular blood supply. 4D-ELF thus may be able to be used as a field scanning technique, to better risk stratify Barrett's patients and also to assess response to various ablative techniques.[29]

BARRETT'S ESOPHAGUS—THERAPY

Flexible endoscopy will evolve over the next decade to become modern operative flexible endoscopy with the advent of advanced tissue resection and other complex endoscopic techniques and maneuvers. One can anticipate a new generation of endoscopes and endosurgical tools, through the scope triangulating instruments and robotic multipronged arms that will allow full thickness resection, anastomosis, wound closure and sewing. Specifically, as applied to the stomach and esophagus, one can anticipate routine removal of tumors and possible nodal dissection that would mimic surgical results. These techniques will build on current efforts surrounding endoscopic mucosal resection (eg, cap-band technique) and submucosal dissection using presently available carbon dioxide insufflation and dissection needles, and en bloc resections using insulation-tipped diathermic knives.[30] It should be noted that in many respects, current endoscopic techniques are already comparable to conventional surgery. Moving forward, there will be significant cost and safety advantages as endoscopic approaches are routinely applied to existing surgical lesions.

Existing ablative techniques also will continue to be applied. Based on the multicenter, randomized, controlled trial of Halo radiofrequency ablation (RFA) recently published in the *New England Journal of Medicine*, RFA has become the standard endoscopic approach to treating Barrett's esophagus with high-grade dysplasia or low-grade dysplasia, in conjunction with endoscopic mucosal resection for nodularity.[31] In this seminal article, in an intention-to-treat analysis, among patients with low-grade dysplasia, complete eradication of dysplasia occurred in 90.5% of those in the ablation group, compared with 22.7% of those in the control group ($P<.001$). In patients with Barrett's high-grade dysplasia, complete eradication was achieved an 81.0% of those in the ablation group compared with 19% of those in the control group ($P<.001$). There was statistically significantly less disease progression in the ablation group (3.6% vs 16.3%; $P<.03$) and significantly fewer cancers (1.2% vs 9.3%; $P = .045$).[31] Comparable results also were obtained in another multicenter, community-based registry study of Barrett's esophagus and high-grade dysplasia, demonstrating that the Halo RFA technique is widely applicable to the general GI community.[32]

This technique also has been demonstrated in multiple clinical trials to be safe and highly effective for the treatment of Barrett's metaplasia. In the *New England Journal of Medicine* article, 77.4% of patients in the ablation group had complete endoscopic and histologic eradication of intestinal metaplasia as compared with 2.3% of those in the control group ($P<.001$). It is highly likely, that going forward, RFA endoscopic ablation will be applied routinely to nondysplastic Barrett's esophagus because of its excellent safety and efficacy record, low Barrett's recurrence rate (<5% at 2 years)[33] and demonstrable cost-effectiveness compared with serial endoscopic surveillance.[34]

Although currently out of favor because of high stricture rates, phototoxicity, and unpredictable response, photodynamic therapy techniques may improve in the future as newer agents become available that will more reliably limit depth of injury and avoid phototoxicity. The ability to predict response to photodynamic therapy also will improve as genetic abnormalities that predispose patients to failure are identified.[35] Other endoscopic ablative techniques also will continue to be developed and applied.

One potential new development is the advent of a device with tiny silicon chips containing wells of drugs or other materials to potentially reverse Barrett's histology. This device can be implanted in a patient to overlay the area with Barrett's esophagus. Once implanted in a patient, the device or the drugs can be activated, supplying either repeated bursts of environmental injury such as radiofrequency ablation or releasing drugs to reverse Barrett's histology or treat dysplasia. Drug-coated stents also could achieve a similar effect. It additionally is possible that inducible pluripotent stem cells could be applied to the area of Barrett's esophagus to achieve Barrett's reversal.

ESOPHAGEAL MOTILITY DISORDERS

There may be revolutionary new approaches to disorders of esophageal motility in the future. Higher resolution manometry systems will allow for better topographic and spatial resolution of esophageal swallowing disorders. New submucosal probes with either chromographic or neurosensory detectors may allow for better determination of the mix of expiratory versus inhibitory neurons in various regions of the esophagus. Esophageal motility is determined largely by the ratio of excitatory input versus inhibitory input, and by the timing and relaxation of these signals. Direct measurement of these neural influences may help improve diagnosis of esophageal motility, and drugs or agents delivered directly to the submucosa or muscle may help improve any physiologic defects.[36]

SUMMARY

The ability to manipulate matter at less than a billionth of a meter, the dramatic advancements in biology, physics and genetics, and the coming revolution in optics will completely transform endoscopic esophageal diagnosis and therapy in the coming years. These developments hold enormous promise for gastroenterologists, but also will be potentially disruptive for current practitioners as new technologies expand the roles of other medical providers, and current practice patterns shift. It is quite likely for example, that light microscopy and histology will be largely replaced by newer, highly accurate, optical imaging systems, thus disrupting the current practice of pathology. Much of current diagnostic endoscopic practice may be taken over by primary care and midlevel providers, as gastroenterologists shift to supervisory roles and move on to higher-level therapeutic and endosurgical techniques. It is also highly likely that current gastroenterology training programs will quickly evolve to some type of hybrid GI-surgical-radiology training to accommodate rapid shifts in technology. These are only some of the dramatic changes to come in the future; certainly there will be many others. The only constant one can assume will be the continuous search for improved diagnosis, therapy, and patient outcomes. That will never change.

REFERENCES

1. Available at: http://www.avantismedical.com. Accessed June 15, 2009.
2. Sandrasegaran K, Maglinte D, Jennings S, et al. Capsule endoscopy and imaging tests in the elective investigation of small bowel disease. Clin Radiol 2008;63(6):712–23.
3. Calabrese C, Bortolotti M, Fabbri A, et al. Reversibility of GERD ultrastructural alterations and relief of symptoms after omeprazole treatment. Am J Gastroenterol 2005;100:537–42.
4. Caviglia R, Ribolsi M, Maggiano N, et al. Dilated intercellular spaces of esophageal epithelium in nonerosive reflux disease patients with physiological esophageal acid exposure. Am J Gastroenterol 2005;100:543–8.
5. Kwiatek M, Hirano I, Kahrilas P, et al. Increased esophagogastric junction distensibility in GERD patients assessed with the endoscopically placed functional luminal imaging probe (EndoFLIP) [abstract]. Gastroenterology 2008;134(4):A591.
6. Pandolfino J, Kahrilas P. American Gastroenterological Association medical position statement: clinical use of esophageal manometry. Gastroenterology 2005; 128:207–24.
7. Hill L, Kozarek R, Kraemer SJM, et al. The gastroesophageal flap valve: in vitro and in vivo observations. Gastrointest Endosc 1996;44(5):541–7.
8. Hockenmeyer D, Soldner F, Cook E, et al. A drug-inducible system for direct reprogramming of human somatic cells to pluripotency. Cell Stem Cell 2008; 3(3):346–53.
9. Ganz R, Fallon E, Wittchow T, et al. A new injectable agent for the treatment of GERD: results of the durasphere pilot trial. Gastrointest Endosc 2009;69(2): 318–23.

10. Cadiere GB, Buset M, Muls V, et al. Antireflux transoral incisionless fundoplication using esophyx: 12-month results of a prospective multicenter study. World J Surg 2008;32(8):1676–88.

11. Ganz R, Gostout C, Berg T, et al. Use of an artificial sphincter for the treatment of GERD—a feasibility study. Gastrointest Endosc 2008;67:287–94.

12. Bonavina L, Saino GI, Lipham J, et al. Magnetic augmentation of the lower esophageal sphincter: results of a feasibility clinical trial. J Gastrointest Surg 2008; 12(12):2133–40.

13. Furuta GT, Liacouras CA, Collins MH, et al. Eosinophilic esophagitis in children and adults: a systematic review and consensus recommendations for diagnosis and treatment. Gastroenterology 2007;133(4):1342–63.

14. Odze R. Pathology of eosinophilic esophagitis: what the clinician needs to know. Am J Gastroenterol 2008;104:485–90.

15. Gonsalves N, Dellon R, Aderoju G, et al. Eosinophilic esophagitis: the newest esophageal inflammatory disease. Gastrointest Endosc 2006;64:313–9.

16. Konikoff MR, Noel RJ, Blanchard C, et al. A randomized, double-blind, placebo-controlled trial of fluticasone propionate for pediatric eosinophilic esophagitis. Gastroenterology 2006;131:1381–91.

17. Bollschweiler E, Wolfgarten E, Gartshow C, et al. Demographic variation in the rising incidence of esophageal adenocarcinoma in white males. Cancer 2001; 92(3):549–55.

18. Kraft P, Hunter DJ. Genetic risk prediction—are we there yet? N Engl J Med 2009; 360(17):1701–3.

19. Montgomery E, Bronner M, Goldblum J, et al. Reproducibility of the diagnosis of dysplasia in Barrett esophagus. Hum Pathol 2001;32(4):368–78.

20. Anagnostopoulos GK, Yao K, Hawkey C, et al. High-resolution endoscopy with narrow band imaging in patients with Barrett's esophagus. Gastrointest Endosc 2006;63:130–6.

21. Wolfsen H, Crook J, Krishna M, et al. Prospective, controlled tandem endoscopy study of narrow band imaging for dysplasia detection in Barrett's esophagus. Gastroenterology 2008;135:24–31.

22. Kiesslich R, Gossner L, Goetz M, et al. In vivo histology of Barrett's esophagus and associated neoplasia by confocal laser endomicroscopy. Clin Gastroenterol Hepatol 2006;4:979–87.

23. Hsiung PL, Hardy J, Friedland S, et al. Detection of colonic dysplasia in vivo using a targeted heptapeptide and confocal microendoscopy. Nat Med 2008;14(4): 454–8.

24. Evans JA, Poneros JM, Bouma BE, et al. Optical coherence tomography to identify intramucosal carcinoma and high-grade dysplasia in Barrett's esophagus. Clin Gastroenterol Hepatol 2006;4:38–43.

25. Wax A, Zhu Y, Terry N, et al. Label-free nuclear morphology measurements of dysplasia in the Egda rat model using angle-resolved low coherence interferometry [abstract]. Gastroenterology 2009;136:AB777.

26. Wallace MB, Wax A, Roberts DN, et al. Reflectance spectroscopy. Gastrointest Endosc Clin N Am 2009;19(2):233–42.

27. Curvers WL, Singh R, Wong-Kee Song LM, et al. Endoscopic trimodal imaging for detection of early neoplasia in Barrett's esophagus. Gut 2008;57: 167–72.

28. Roy H, Gomes A, Turzhitsky V, et al. Spectroscopic microvascular blood detection from the endoscopically normal colonic mucosa: biomarker for neoplasia risk. Gastroenterology 2008;135:1069–78.

29. Buchner A, Wallace MB. Novel endoscopic approaches in detecting colorectal neoplasia: macroscopes, microscopes, and metal detectors. Gastroenterology 2008;135:1035–7.
30. Repici A. Endoscopic submucosal dissection: established, or still needs improving? Gastrointest Endosc 2009;69(1):16–8.
31. Shaheen N, Sharma P, Overholt BF, et al. Radiofrequency ablation in Barrett's esophagus with dysplasia. N Engl J Med 2009;360:2277–88.
32. Ganz R, Overholt BF, Sharma VK, et al. Circumferential ablation of Barrett's esophagus that contains high-grade dysplasia: a US multicenter registry. Gastrointest Endosc 2008;68(1):35–40.
33. Shaheen N, Sharma P, Overholt BF, et al. How durable is the reversion to neosquamous epithelium in subjects undergoing radiofrequency ablation for dysplastic Barrett's esophagus? Two-year follow-up of the aim–dysplasia randomized sham-controlled trial [abstract]. Gastroenterology 2009;136:AB1039.
34. Inadomi JM, Somsouk M, Madanick RD, et al. A cost-utility analysis of ablative therapy for Barrett's esophagus. Gastroenterology 2009;136(7):2101–14.
35. Prasad G, Wang K, Halling K, et al. Utility of biomarkers in prediction of response to ablative therapy in Barrett's esophagus. Gastroenterology 2008;135(2):370–9.
36. Sumiyama K, Tajiri H, Kato F, et al. Pilot study for in vivo cellular imaging of the muscularis propria and ex vivo molecular imaging of myenteric neurons. Gastrointest Endosc 2009;69(6):1129–34.

Index

Note: Page numbers of article titles are in **boldface** type.

A

Adenocarcinoma
  esophageal, Barrett esophagus progression to, risk factors for, 2–3
  prevention of, 4
ALA. See *Aminolevulinic acid (ALA).*
Aminolevulinic acid (ALA), 41–42
Atofluorescence imaging, in detection of esophageal dysplasia and carcinoma, 19

B

BARD EndoCinch, in GERD management, 94
Barrett esophagus, 2
  colon adenoma/CRC vs., 3–4
  described, 55–56, 75
  diagnosis of, future of, 151–155
  endoscopic treatment of, rationale for, 4–6
  esophageal dysplasia and carcinoma in, endoscopic therapy using RFA for, **55–74.**
    See also *Radiofrequency ablation (RFA), for esophageal dysplasia and carcinoma in Barrett esophagus, endoscopic therapy using.*
  imaging for, future of, 20–21
  progression to dysplasia, risk factors for, 2–3
  progression to esophageal adenocarcinoma, risk factors for, 2–3
  risk stratification for, 151–155
  treatment of, future of, 155–156
  with or without dysplasia, cryotherapy for, results of, 81–82
Barrett esophagus/HGD, photodynamic therapy for, 36–38
Barrett mucosa, with HGD in distal esophagus and cardia, complete removal of, EMR and ESD in, 32–33
Biomarker(s), PDT and, 43–46
Biopsy, pleural, 130

C

Cancer(s), esophageal
  cryotherapy for, results of, 82–83
  described, 103–104
  endoprevention of, 1–2
Cap-fitted endoscope, EMR using, for esophageal dysplasia and carcinoma, 26–29
Chromoendoscopy, in detection of esophageal dysplasia and carcinoma, 12–13
Colon adenoma/CRC, Barrett esophagus/esophageal adenocarcinoma vs., 3–4
Colon and rectal carcinoma (CRC)
  Barrett esophagus/esophageal adenocarcinoma vs., 3–4
  prevention of, 4

Gastrointest Endoscopy Clin N Am 20 (2010) 161–167
doi:10.1016/S1052-5157(09)00132-9
1052-5157/09/$ – see front matter © 2010 Elsevier Inc. All rights reserved.

Moving?

Make sure your subscription moves with you!

To notify us of your new address, find your **Clinics Account Number** (located on your mailing label above your name), and contact customer service at:

Email: journalscustomerservice-usa@elsevier.com

800-654-2452 (subscribers in the U.S. & Canada)
314-447-8871 (subscribers outside of the U.S. & Canada)

Fax number: 314-447-8029

Elsevier Health Sciences Division
Subscription Customer Service
3251 Riverport Lane
Maryland Heights, MO 63043

*To ensure uninterrupted delivery of your subscription, please notify us at least 4 weeks in advance of move.

Printed and bound by CPI Group (UK) Ltd, Croydon, CR0 4YY

03/10/2024

01040454-0012